Antioxidants *against* Cancer

OTHER BOOKS BY RALPH W. MOSS, PHD

Herbs Against Cancer

Alternative Medicine Online

Questioning Chemotherapy

Cancer Therapy

The Cancer Industry

Free Radical: Albert Szent-Gyorgyi
and the Battle Over Vitamin C

Caring
(with Annette Swackhamer, RN)

A Real Choice

An Alternative Approach to Allergies
(with Theron G. Randolph, MD)

The Cancer Syndrome

Antioxidants *against* Cancer

Ralph W. Moss, PhD

Equinox Press, Inc.

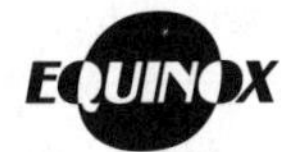

Manufactured in the United States of America by
Equinox Press
P.O. Box 8183
State College, PA 16803

Second Printing 2002
Cover and book design by Martha Bunim

Library of Congress Cataloging-in-Publication Data
Moss, Ralph W.
Antioxidants against cancer / Ralph W. Moss
p. cm.
Includes bibliographical references
ISBN 1-881025-28-47
1. Cancer--Chemoprevention. 2. Antioxidants--Therapeutic use.
3. Cancer--Diet therapy. I. Title.

RC268.15 .M67 2000
616.99'406--dc21 99-057585

Table of Contents

Note to Reader

1. The Power of Antioxidants

"What can I do to prevent cancer?"

Of the many questions that I receive every day, this is the most frequent and most urgent. It comes from people who have had cancer and from those who have watched friends and relatives struggle with this disease. It comes from people of every class, occupation, and age. Cancer is frightening, debilitating, and expensive. It disrupts and destroys lives, careers, whole families. No one is immune.

The good news is that because of scientific knowledge gained in the last decade, it is possible for individuals to reduce their risk of many kinds of cancers. The key to risk reduction is diet, food supplements, avoidance of carcinogens, and other life style improvements. Environmental factors may cause up to 70 percent of all cancers. Even cancers caused by genetic defects can be helped by antioxidants.

Another question is, **"How can I prevent the side effects of surgery, radiation, and chemotherapy?"** Patients want to minimize the damage to their blood and bone marrow, the hair loss, mouth sores, and other miseries that sometimes make radiation and chemotherapy a nightmare. It is my firm belief that antioxidants can be used by patients undergoing conventional treatments such as radiation and chemotherapy. **Antioxidants can be very helpful in reducing side effects.**

Once patients have completed conventional therapy, is there anything they can do to speed their recovery? The answer is Yes! **Antioxidants can stimulate the body's innate healing powers and restore wellness.**

In addition to improving one's diet, one should stop using tobacco and other harmful substances, increase physical activity and exercise, avoid unnecessary X rays, and maintain an optimistic mental attitude. These are all very important in preventing cancer.

The term "antioxidant" was coined in the 1920s to denote any substance that fought rust, or other forms of oxidation. Oxygen-containing compounds give rise to molecules called "free radicals." In the body, free radicals can set off little chain reactions that wreak havoc.

Scientific work over the last few decades has shown that free radicals can also damage genetic material, lipids (fats), or proteins. (150) They are also believed to be responsible for many of the effects of aging and for diseases such as cancer. Even cancers that were once thought to be caused by mechanical injury (such as asbestos-caused mesothelioma) now turn out to have a free radical component. (323)

In the last decade, research on antioxidants has come to the fore as an important component of any anticancer program. Antioxidants fight cancer at every level and every stage. Along with other plant-based nutrients, they are our first and strongest defense against cancers of many kinds.

Attitudes of Doctors

Thousands of scientific articles point to the power of antioxidants, yet many doctors are not taught about this in medical school. Others may know about this exciting development but shy away from it because they fear peer pressure or stigmatization. And all too often, doctors respond to positive reports with a warning that patients should not take food supplements.

The conventional line is that the research is promising, but there just isn't enough data on which to base firm conclusions. But doctors and people in general often make decisions in the absence of certainty. Consider these words of Richard Horton, M.D., the editor-in-chief of the *Lancet*, in a 1998 editorial on the "Precautionary Principle":

Dr. Horton's Precautionary Principle

"We must act on facts," Dr. Horton wrote, "and on the most accurate interpretation of them, using the best scientific information. That does not mean that we must sit back until we have 100 percent evidence about everything. When the state of the health of the people is at stake...we should be prepared to take action to diminish those risks even when the scientific knowledge is not conclusive...." (173)

This same Precautionary Principle has been applied by some doctors to make recommendations on supplements. (129) The cost of inaction is tremendous, and the "health of the people" is definitely at stake. At the same time, I strongly believe in science and all the recommendations in this book are based on scientific findings.

The Cost of Inaction

According to the World Health Organization, there were 10 million new cases of cancer in 1996, and by the year 2001 they predict a yearly total of 14.7 million. These numbers are so huge that the suffering they imply is incomprehensible.

In the United States, there are about 1.2 million new cases and over 560,000 deaths from cancer every year. Yet progress in treatment and prevention has been painfully slow. The mortality rate in 1994 was six percent higher than in 1970. And although there has been a slight downturn since then (probably due to smoking cessation), it is not enough to change a generally bleak picture: every other man and every third woman in the United States is now slated to get cancer—unless they do something dramatic to change that. The purpose of this book is to help you keep out of the cancer record books.

Certainly, few medical interventions can have less risk than eating a diet high in antioxidants. We are not talking about taking arsenic here, but about brightly colored fruits and vegetables, as well as their concentrated extracts. Yet many physicians draw the line when you discuss antioxidants and say, "Much too risky. Not enough known."

No wonder that laypeople are turning to books, magazines, and Websites for information on antioxidants, and that many patients hesitate to even discuss questions of nutrition with their doctor. Patients are becoming more educated (sometimes more educated than their doctors!) and more empowered.

Cancer patients cannot wait for some hypothetical state of complete knowledge. **They must make decisions based on today's knowledge.** It is my privilege to summarize and interpret the data that already exists and to show you how I draw my conclusions. But I also give you enough information to make up your own mind.

Although the focus of this book is on cancer, antioxidants are also important in the prevention of heart attacks, strokes, macular degeneration of the eye, and about one hundred other illnesses associated with aging. Thus, the reasons for including antioxidant-rich foods and supplements in your daily routine goes far beyond the question of cancer.

It is also crucial to realize that antioxidants are just one part of a cancer prevention picture. There are other parts, including beneficial herbs, fatty acids, algae, mushrooms, etc., whose primary mode of action may not be due to antioxidation. You will find an abundance of resources on these topics at my website, **cancerdecisions.com.**

Five a Day

The National Cancer Institute recommends that people eat five portions of fruits and vegetables per day. Here is official recognition of the power of antioxidants. There's no question that this five a day campaign is one of the best things NCI has ever done. However, there are several limitations. There is very little publicity for this campaign; five one-half cup portions per day may not be enough to get the maximum effect; and most importantly, it is impossible or impractical for most people to get all their nutrients through food alone. Supplementation is necessary.

In fact, few people actually get the five portions of fruits and vegetables per day that NCI recommends. The average in 1995 was 3.4 servings per day for adults, while kids got only 25 percent of the recommended vegetable servings per day. (427) This persistent lack of vital nutrients will affect the future of these children and of our society.

It is becoming increasingly obvious that food supplementation is necessary to prevent cancer and other diseases. The prestigious Institute of Medicine (IOM) of the National Academy of Sciences in 1998 called for supplementation with folic acid and vitamin B12. The *Berkeley Wellness Letter* has increased its recommendation for both vitamin C and E to daily amounts that are only practical to achieve through supplementation. The *Journal of the American Medical Association* and other medical journals are now talking openly about higher doses.

So perhaps we shall see the day when studies showing that antioxidants prevent cancer are followed by the recommendation, "Try adding these to your diet!"

2. *Antioxidants as Cancer Therapy*

Some patients try to find ways of treating their cancer after conventional methods have failed. Some try to avoid surgery, radiation, and chemotherapy in the first place.

Many of us have heard stories of people who have employed antioxidants, often in high doses, and achieved remissions of their cancers. Dozens of practitioners use antioxidants as part of their unconventional treatment programs. **Such treatments are promising but not proven.**

Most of them derive from the program advocated by Linus Pauling, Ph.D., and carried out by his Scottish colleague, Ewan Cameron, M.D. I have written about Dr. Pauling's struggles in my book, *The Cancer Industry*. Many have heard that this treatment was tested at the Mayo Clinic and found wanting. (288) However, there are reasons to believe the test was not carried out fairly. Others besides myself have called for further investigation of this method. (182)

The charge is sometimes made that alternative doctors are remiss in not carrying out randomized clinical trials (RCTs) to prove the effectiveness of antioxidants as cancer therapy. A clinical trial involves testing in human beings. In a randomized trial, patients are assigned to different treatment regimens, and the two or more groups are then compared. It is not a simple matter to arrange and then carry out clinical trials. It requires many resources, such as money and access to suitable patients.

We shall point out positive human clinical studies in the course of this book. Most of these deal with individual agents. Here are several studies in which a combination of high-dose antioxidants worked very well.

High-Dose Antioxidants with BCG for Bladder Cancer

A double-blind clinical trial on the use of high-dose antioxidants as a treatment for bladder cancer turned out highly positive. Dr. David L. Lamm and colleagues at the West Virginia School of Medicine treated 65 patients with bladder cancer with a standard treatment called BCG. Thirty patients were given small doses of antioxidants (at the low government-approved RDA levels) while thirty-five patients were given megadoses. (224)

The megadose levels were as follows:

Supplement	*Amount Given Daily*
Vitamin C	2,000 milligrams
Vitamin A	40,000 international units
Vitamin B6	100 milligrams
Vitamin E	400 international units
Zinc	90 milligrams

Bladder cancer frequently recurs. But ten months after starting the program, the rate of recurrence in the megadose group began to fall. At five years, the rate of recurrence in the megadose group was 41 percent, compared with 91 percent in those receiving the small RDA doses.

By the end of the study, 24 out of 30 patients in the low-dose group had suffered recurrences, while just 14 out of 35 in the high-dose group had new tumors. **In other words, megadoses of antioxidants reduced one's chances of a recurrence of bladder cancer in half.** (224)

This is precisely the kind of study that the medical establishment has demanded as proof of the benefits of megadose antioxidant therapy.

Are Megadoses Better than RDA Doses?

In Greece, scientists gave either low or high doses of combinations of vitamins to rats with experimentally induced sarcomas. This was a mixture of vitamins C and E, selenium and another substance called 2-MPG. The low dose combination failed to exert any beneficial effect on the survival of the animals. In fact, such animals had more lung tumors. But the high-dose group had a significant prolongation in survival. There was a complete remission of tumors in 16.8 percent of the animals. The authors concluded that megadoses of these substances are probably needed in to achieve "a sufficient prevention and treatment of malignant diseases." (109)

Long Beach Multivitamin Trial

In a 1996 clinical study of high-dose antioxidants, doctors at the Long Beach Veterans' Administration hospital and the University of California, Irvine, reached similar conclusions. Ten patients with various cancers (including non-Hodgkin's lymphoma, breast, esophageal, lung, head-and-neck, colon and choriocarcinoma) were given a variety of chemotherapy regimens. These included the CHOP regimen, carboplatin, Adriamycin,

5-FU, VP-16, and others.

Before such toxic treatments, patients were given high doses of the antioxidant vitamins A, C, and E, as well as the mineral selenium. When the patients received these nutrients their white blood cell (neutrophil) count increased by nearly 300 percent! Nine out of ten patients whose blood scores had plummeted in earlier courses of drugs achieved stable levels when they were given high-dose antioxidants. (446)

Note: you should not take high doses of fat-soluble vitamins, such as A and E, unless under a doctor's care, since they can accumulate in the body and become toxic.

After these studies were done, it was business as usual in the world of conventional cancer treatment. No follow-up studies were done and few cancer patients have ever heard about it. Only holistic physicians such as Robert Atkins, M.D. have publicized this information in their books and lectures to bolster patients' chances of success in beating cancer. (19)

3. Foods and Antioxidants

Hopefully, you now want to enlist antioxidants in your own personal fight to prevent or treat cancer. What is the best way to get these powerful nutrients into your system? Should you attempt to get all your antioxidants from your food or should you take food supplements? Here are the benefits of getting antioxidants from food:

- Foods contain many antioxidants, some of which may not even be known to science yet. There are hundreds of carotenoids alone.
- Foods are a dependable source, and you won't go wrong if you pick fresh, deeply colored, organic produce.
- Foods are an economical way of getting antioxidants. You have to eat, and so you might as well choose foods rich in health-giving factors.
- Science shows a very strong correlation between diets high in antioxidants and cancer prevention.

Benefits of Supplements

Food is the mainstay of your antioxidant program. But I strongly believe that it is necessary to take supplements in addition to foods in order to get the maximum benefit. Some critics claim that the supplements you buy in the health food store are completely unreliable. This is an exaggeration. The large vitamin and mineral suppliers generally conform to "USP" standards, and their products are reliable. But herbs and food extracts, such as concentrated berry supplements, vary considerably in their ingredients and potency, as we shall see.

Lately, the National Nutritional Foods Association (NNFA), has instituted a "TruLabel program." Under this program, companies pay for an independent laboratory to test their products at random. If a test reveals that a product or ingredient is deficient, the member company is then contacted and given a brief period to correct the problem. Any company that then fails to comply is expelled from membership in NNFA, and is unable to exhibit at their shows. The situation is evolving towards greater reliability for health food products in general.

Until recently, we had no way to know just how potent a formula was or how one compared with another. In the early 1990s, however, Dr. Guohua Cao and his colleagues came up with an ingenious solution. They created a standardized test for measuring and comparing various foods for their antioxidant power. (59) This is the Oxygen Radical Absorbance Capacity (or ORAC) test.

The ORAC test compares the antioxidant power of various samples, which can be foods, supplements, or even bodily fluids. Each substance tested is compared to the power in a standardized amount of vitamin E.

Antioxidant Values of Selected Fruits and Vegetables

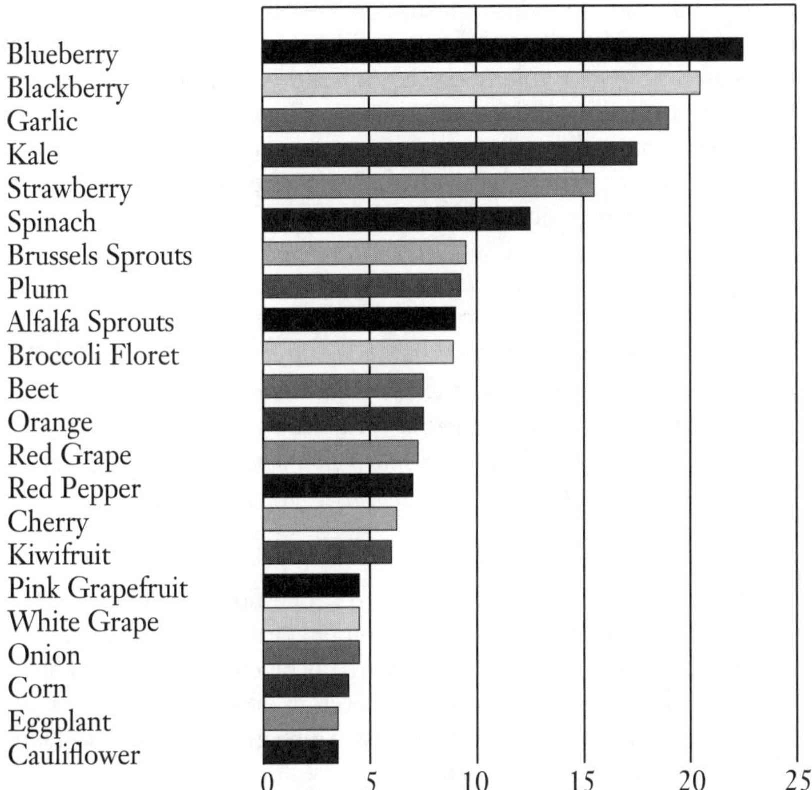

Information reprinted with permission of Dr. Ronald Prior, USDA.

In 1994, Dr. Cao came to work with Dr. Ronald Prior at the USDA laboratory at Tufts University, Boston, and they turned their attention to foods thought to be high in antioxidants. While in the past people tended to view all colorful vegetables as equally beneficial, in these USDA tests a few foods jumped out as the superstars of antioxidants. Leading the pack was the wild blueberry.

Scientists attributed its superior power to "anthocyanins" and other antioxidants found particularly in berries. The term "anthocyanin" comes from two Greek words meaning "blue" and "plant"; they are responsible for the intense blue and red pigments of blueberries, raspberries and strawberries. (44) Close behind the berries were garlic and kale. Spinach, Brussels sprouts, plums, alfalfa sprouts, broccoli, beets, oranges, red grapes, red peppers, cherries, kiwis, and pink grapefruits also contained significant amounts of antioxidants.

White grapes, onions, corn, eggplant, and cauliflower all had some, although only about one-fifth the amount contained in the dark berries.

Dr. Cao and his colleagues also studied the effect of foods high in ORACs on the blood of volunteers. Eight healthy but elderly women were given meals with measured amounts of foods. The amount of antioxidants in the blood jumped up after a meal supplemented with strawberry or spinach extracts, or with red wine. In fact, a large portion of strawberry or spinach was shown to equal 1,250 milligrams of vitamin C in terms of antioxidant power. (59)

In an interesting side note, the antioxidant level of people's blood increases significantly after the consumption of any meal. Why should this be? Tufts scientists speculate that we have an innate antioxidant ability, which swings into action when we eat because the body knows that the act of digestion itself generates free radicals.

How do fruits and fruit juices compare? The Boston scientists looked at the antioxidant power of a dozen commonly eaten fruits and five commercial fruit juices. In this test, from which blueberries were excluded, strawberries had the highest score, followed in order by plums, oranges, red grapes, kiwi fruit, pink grapefruits, white grapes, bananas, apples, tomatoes, pears, and honeydew melon.

Most of the antioxidant power of these fruits was located in the juice portion, while the pulp contributed few antioxidants (although it contains fiber and other useful things). Among the commercial fruit juices, grape juice had the highest antioxidant power, followed by grapefruit, tomato, orange, and apple juice.

Although not tested, a logical choice for both adults and children are those increasingly popular drinks made up of cranberry, grape, raspberry, and apple juices. Look for the kind that is 100 percent juice, or else you will wind up paying for a lot of sugar, corn sweetener, and water.

Fruit of the Year

Tufts scientists also found that antioxidant-rich foods, such as blueberries, help to halt the aging process. Rats given blueberry extracts showed fewer of the mental deficits that are characteristic of aging. (189)

There has been an avalanche of good publicity on the health benefits of blueberries. Dr. Prior confessed that he has added blueberries to his regular diet. In December, 1998, *Eating Well* magazine named the blueberry "Fruit of the Year," and in June, 1999, *Prevention* dubbed it the Miracle Berry.

"If you add one food to your diet this year, make it blueberries," said *Prevention's* Nutrition Editor. According to her, blueberries are the **"single most ferocious food in the supermarket at halting the forces that age you."**

In 1998, scientists at Rutgers University in New Jersey showed that blueberries, like cranberries, contain substances that prevent the *E. coli* bacteria from adhering to the walls of the urinary tract and causing troublesome urinary tract infections (UTIs). (174)

In the summer in Maine, I avail myself of every opportunity to eat fresh blueberries. I am fortunate, since there are abandoned blueberry fields within walking distance of my house, and there is usually plenty of fruit for the taking. I also seek out the organic producers in my area, stock up on blueberries while they are plentiful, and freeze them for the berryless months ahead. The news that blueberries are healthful was greeted with a knew-it-all-along smile by my Downeast neighbors.

Those Amazing Teas

Teas, both the black and green varieties, have much higher antioxidant values than any vegetables. Chemicals named catechins in green tea are powerful anticancer agents.

Japanese scientists treated rats with a dose of a carcinogen. They then placed some of the rats on a diet containing various antioxidants, including green tea catechins. The difference in survival between the treated and the untreated groups was startling. Where only a third of the rats receiving just the ordinary diet were alive at the end of the experiment, **an extraordinary 93.8 percent of the rats receiving green tea catechins were still alive!** (170)

By dry weight, both green and black tea had fantastically high levels of antioxidants, higher than any other plants tested, as we have said. But of course we don't normally *eat* tea. Do brewed teas give us the benefit of these high levels?

The scientists tested both green and black tea by brewing them in boiling water. And indeed, about 84 percent of the total antioxidant activity of the tea emerged within the first 5 minutes of brewing. An additional 13 percent was extracted in the following 5 minutes. This means that tea should be brewed for about 10 minutes for maximum antioxidant value, although 5 minutes also yields a potent brew.

Five-minute tea gave an ORAC score of 8.31. So its antioxidant capacity is comparable to fruit juices, which range from 1.6 up to 15. At these levels, the consumption of a five-ounce cup of tea could make a significant contribution to your daily antioxidant intake.

And, I might add, tea is one of the great food bargains of all time, costing a fraction of the cost of the equivalent amount of fruit juices.

On the Variability of Supplements

At this moment, I would not generally recommend berry supplements, and here's why. While foods have some variability in their antioxidant power, there are tremendous differences in the potency of supplements containing berry extracts.

In the summer of 1999, Tufts scientists published a paper on the variability of antioxidants in food supplements. They looked at 46 different commercial preparations, most of which were derived from berries known to be high in antioxidant power, including the European bilberry, cranberry, chokeberry, and elderberry. In these samples, some brands had an extraordinary one-thousand times more antioxidants than the others. Similarly, when they looked at celebrated sources of antioxidants such as pine bark and grape seed extracts, they also found a huge variation in potency. Some of these products were 400 times more powerful than others.

The results from this study show that better quality control of antioxidants is needed before one can make a recommendation about taking a particular brand of supplements. **You should check with your local health food store owner for advice on the best brands.** Also see the excellent new Website, www.consumerlabs.com for evaluations.

Optimum Health

Just how much antioxidant power do you need to promote optimum health? In the U.S., the average ORAC intake from fruits and vegetables is around 1,200 per day. People who average five fruit and vegetable servings per day boost their intake to about 1,640. **However, individuals who deliberately choose a diet that is high in the most powerful fruits and vegetables can raise this fourfold, to 6,000 per day. Attaining this many antioxidants in the diet is a goal that everyone should aspire to.**

Grapes and Wine

Red grapes always score high on the antioxidant charts. This is most likely due to the presence of an intriguing substance called resveratrol. Resveratrol is an antioxidant found in many foods, but most abundantly in peanuts and red grapes.

Red wine from cold climates (such as France) is a particularly good source of resveratrol. It is less concentrated in red wines from warmer climes such as California, Italy, Spain, or Portugal.

Studies from the University of Illinois have shown that the number of early breast lesions and skin cancers in mice dropped dramatically when they were given high doses of resveratrol. (183)

Whether or not to drink wine, however, involves a number of factors. Some people are prone to alcoholism, and need to avoid alcoholic beverages. Others suffer from allergic reactions to the sulfites in wine, especially red wine. People with heart arrhythmias or prostate problems might also find their conditions exacerbated by strong wines.

There is also some fear that alcohol promotes breast cancer, although I do not find the data for this compelling. But if you can and do enjoy wine, get some French red wine and enjoy from as little as two glasses per week to as many as two per day. Remember that resveratrol disappears from an uncorked bottle of wine at room temperature in a day, but will last about a week in the refrigerator.

To summarize: Colorful fruits and vegetables are a fantastic source of potent antioxidants. The most powerful fruits are the berries, particularly wild blueberries. Berry-containing juices are a convenient and economical way to obtain their health benefits. Black, and especially, green teas are wonderfully beneficial as they are also extremely high in antioxidant power. Grapes, grape juice and red wine are also very worthwhile sources of antioxidants. One should also eat the seeds in grapes (see chapter 14). We cannot recommend any particular brands of berry extracts at this time, since they fluctuate greatly in strength and purity.

4. Antioxidants and Conventional Therapies

Should cancer patients take antioxidants during conventional treatments such as surgery, radiation, and chemotherapy? Surveys show that many patients are doing just that, although they often keep quiet about it because they believe that their oncologist will not be sympathetic. This is not necessarily the case: I believe the oncology profession is confused and divided on this issue.

In fact, when patients at M.D. Anderson Cancer Center in Houston discussed alternative medicine with their oncologists, the reaction was mixed: most doctors were either neutral or encouraged such use. Only 17 percent warned against potential risks, while a mere 2.1 percent actively discouraged the use of nonconventional approaches. (373)

The vocal minority who oppose food supplements tend to dominate the discussion, but do not necessarily reflect the opinion of most oncologists. Test out your doctor with a few general questions. If he or she is receptive, share your desire to use antioxidants as part of your overall treatment plan.

Point out to them that the preponderance of data supports the concurrent use of antioxidants and chemotherapy. Give them a copy of this book and encourage them to read it.

Fear of Antioxidants

I do not want to get into a technical discussion here of how antioxidants interact with radiation or chemotherapy. **But some doctors fear that supplements could cancel the effects of their toxic treatments.** This was the basis of a 1999 polemic by a naturopath, Dan Labriola, and oncologist Robert Livingston in the journal *Oncology*. (222)

I don't agree with this. The actual data (which I present throughout this book) overwhelmingly contradicts the idea that antioxidants cancel the effects of toxic treatments. Quite the opposite: almost every experiment on the topic supports the idea that there is synergy, that is, increased benefits when antioxidants and toxic treatments are used together.

Another reason to take supplements is that toxic treatments routinely rob patients of key nutrients. Almost every vitamin, from A to K, has been found to be lacking in some cancer patients after they receive chemotherapy. Plus, cancer itself can sometimes cause deficiencies and malnutrition. One of the reasons for malnutrition is that chemotherapy can cause nausea, vomiting, infection, fever, and a generalized state of anxiety. All of these can contribute to weight loss and the wasting syndrome called cachexia.

Antioxidant supplements can play a role in restoring a cancer patient's nutritional status to normal. So taking supplements is a logical way of returning what was lost due to conventional treatments and disease.

Loss of Antioxidants

The same pattern holds true for radiation therapy. The decline in antioxidants after radiation can be subtle but long-lasting. Many oncologists believe that antioxidants spring back quickly after radiation. Not so.

At Leiden University Medical Center, scientists found that the levels of the antioxidants bilirubin, albumin, and uric acid all remained low for quite a while after radiation, as did the ratio of vitamin E to cholesterol and triglycerides. The Dutch doctors called this "a failure of the antioxidant defense mechanism against oxidative damage" caused by commonly used toxic treatments. (469)

It is very important to bring these antioxidant levels up. Albumin alone is a bellwether of how long a person will live—a "significant independent predictor of survival."(110) Antioxidants in the diet can bolster the body's overall antioxidant levels.

Scientists in Tübingen, Germany, have looked at the levels of vitamins C and E, beta-carotene, etc., before, during, and after high-dose chemotherapy. The drug etoposide significantly increased free radical damage to fats. (223) Beta-carotene levels fell by 50 percent and vitamin E (alpha-tocopherol) levels by 20 percent. (73)

Many other studies could be cited to show that chemotherapy as well as radiation can cause malnutrition and vitamin deficiencies. (97) The symptoms may be masked by the other side effects of treatment or of the cancer itself. Cancer patients, by and large, are not getting back the antioxidants that are taken from them by these highly toxic treatments.

To summarize: Antioxidants do not interfere with radiation or chemotherapy. In fact, they make them easier for the patients to take. I shall have much more to say about the interactions of specific antioxidants with toxic therapies in the following chapters on individual nutrients.

5. Vitamin A

Let us now turn our attention to the dietary antioxidants, which are present in our food and also available as food supplements. These are all non-toxic in reasonable amounts and most are relatively inexpensive. For about one dollar per day you can provide yourself with a powerful antioxidant program to reduce your risk of cancer, as well as many other illnesses. There are few bargains in health care greater than this.

Vitamin A

What is vitamin A? Can it reduce the risk of cancer? What effect does it have on a person who already has the disease? And how does it interact with toxic treatments?

As its position in the alphabet indicates, vitamin A was the first vitamin to be isolated and chemically defined. In its most common form it is called "retinol," and therefore drugs similar to it are called "retinoids."

Vitamin A gives us the ability to see at night. It also fortifies the mucous membranes of the body, which are our first barrier against poisons, microbes, and cancer-causing substances. Some other benefits of vitamin A are protection of the thymus gland (which is vital for immunity) and aid in making proteins. And like many other nutrients, vitamin A is an antioxidant, which can soak up harmful free radicals.

Evidence for a link between vitamin A deficiency and cancer goes back 75 years. In 1926, a Japanese scientist found that lab animals on a vitamin A-deprived diet were more likely to develop cancer than those fed the usual enriched lab chow. Two years later, other scientists extended this finding to human cancers as well. Around the same time, **a Harvard researcher pointed out the similarity between vitamin A-deprived cells and cancer cells.**

In the 1960s, Dr. Wolfgang Scheef of the Janker Clinic, Bonn, began to use extremely high doses of vitamin A as part of his innovative cancer therapy program. (172)

In 1963, vitamin A was shown to prevent and even cure a condition called leukoplakia—which are white and warty patches in the mouth that often precede cancer. Dr. Umberto Saffiotti, who was the dean of vitamin A studies in America, showed that mice could be protected against cancers of the lungs, stomach, gastrointestinal tract, and uterus with vitamin A. **Sometimes the protection was nearly 100 percent complete.** This finding caused considerable excitement. (382a)

In 1971, Dr. Raymond Shamberger of the Cleveland Clinic showed that vitamin A could decrease the number of skin cancers (routinely initiated by chemical carcinogens in the laboratory) by 76 percent. This finding led to the development of vitamin A derivatives to treat skin cancer. Retinoids were found to act as "differentiation agents," an important new category in cancer treatment. Such findings have "generated widespread interest in these agents for cancer treatment and prevention," according to a major cancer textbook. (464)

Animal experiments and population-based studies were begun in the 1970s to test this hypothesis. (107) For example, in 1975, Norwegian scientists found, after correcting for smoking habits, more lung cancer among the men who got the least vitamin A. (37) Other studies strongly supported this concept. (267)

Diet, Nutrition and Cancer

By 1981, there were hundreds of positive reports on vitamin A and cancer in the medical literature. In 1982, the National Academy of Sciences landmark study, *Diet, Nutrition and Cancer*, concluded, "Of the entire collection of chemically diverse substances classified as vitamins, those subsumed under the general term 'vitamin A' are of the greatest current interest in terms of their possible association with the process of carcinogenesis [cancer formation]."

In the early 1980s, a well-known Oxford University researcher, Richard Peto, suggested that a diet high in carrots and similar vegetables could reduce the risk of cancer. "I believe there is now a light at the end of our tunnel in our fight against this disease," he told a conference. (346) He stated there was a 40 percent lower risk of cancer among men who maintained above average consumption of vitamin A than in those who were deficient. Later, these studies were extended to vitamin A's non-toxic relative beta-carotene as well.

At Stockholm's famous Karolinska Hospital, scientists gave healthy subjects vitamin A pills. After a few years, they noted that vitamin A decreased the risk of cancer in these people. They speculated that vitamin A works by trapping cell-damaging free radicals and neutralizing their cancer-causing effects. (421)

In a population-based study, scientists at NCI followed up on nearly 2,500 men over the age of 50 for years. Eighty-four of these men developed cancer of the prostate. The levels of vitamin A in their blood were significantly lower than among the men who did not develop this disease. **In general, the lower the blood level of vitamin A, the greater the risk of developing prostate cancer.** This was the first time that vitamin A and prostate cancer were linked in a large study. (372a)

One hundred and six people with lung cancer volunteered for a dietary study in southwest France. Scientists found low levels of vitamin A and beta-carotene in their diets. This provided fresh evidence that vitamin A had a protective effect against lung cancer. (85)

Dutch scientists also studied the blood levels of vitamin A in 86 patients with cancers of the head and neck. Some of these patients had tumors at other sites as well. Thirty-one percent of the patients with just head-and-neck cancers had low blood levels of vitamin A. But when scientists looked at those patients who had cancer at two sites, the number with low levels of vitamin A leaped to 60 percent. They recommended that patients with head-and-neck tumors be given vitamin A supplements in order to prevent a second tumor from forming. (91)

Study in Polyps

Polyps are abnormal growth in the rectum and colon that may progress to cancer in some people. In 1992, scientists in Bologna, Italy reported that a combination of vitamins A, C, and E could correct abnormalities in the cells of the rectum in people who previously had polyps removed. There was a decrease in the number of premalignant cells in patients who received the three vitamins, compared to patients who received none. (337)

Since it is fat soluble (like vitamins D, E and K), vitamin A can accumulate in the body. It thus can be toxic in high doses. As an interesting side light, the patients in the Bologna study were given relatively high doses of vitamin A—25,000 to 50,000 International Units (IU) per day for months. There were no side effects at this level.

One retinoid often used in cancer therapy is the common acne medication, Accutane (or 13-cis-retinoic acid). Like vitamin A, when taken in excess, it can cause extremely dry skin, chapped lips, eye problems (conjunctivitis) and increased levels of fat in the blood. (337)

Frank L. Meyskens, Jr., M.D., has found that vitamin A-like substances can be beneficial for some kinds of cancer. "I think increasingly, we will find the retinoids in and of themselves will impact the prevention and treatment of cancer," he has said. For example, a rapidly growing kind of skin cancer (keratoacanthoma) responds to Accutane.

In 1985, doctors at M.D. Anderson Cancer Center, Houston, proposed the experimental use of Accutane as a treatment for head-and-neck cancers. In the *New England Journal of Medicine* in 1990, they reported on their positive results. After receiving surgery, radiation therapy, or both, 103 patients were given either Accutane or a placebo (inert sugar pill), which they took daily for 12 months.

The group receiving Accutane had "significantly fewer second primary tumors." After 32 months, only 2 patients (4 percent) in the Accutane group had second primary tumors, compared with 12 (24 percent) in the placebo group. Some of those in the placebo group had multiple cancers appear. Of the 14 second cancers, 13 (or 93 percent) occurred in the head and neck, esophagus or lung, the Houston researchers said.

Daily treatment with high doses of Accutane was effective in preventing second primary tumors in patients who had been treated for squamous-cell carcinoma of the head and neck, although it did not prevent recurrences of the original tumors. (172a)

Another retinoid (transretinoic acid) was applied topically to treat a condition called dysplastic nevi syndrome. This is a mole that can turn into the skin cancer, malignant melanoma.

Some other patients with advanced skin cancers also benefited from this therapy. One patient with 30 skin cancers on his hands was scheduled to have both hands amputated. He showed such tremendous improvement on Accutane that the surgery was canceled and he remained free of the disease for many years.

THE TUMOR VANISHES: Steve Otto is a Washington, D.C. bartender who had cancer of the mouth. Six weeks of radiation and four months of chemotherapy had failed to halt the growth of his tumor. He was then offered a new treatment at Georgetown's Lombardi Cancer Center in Washington, DC: a vitamin A derivative, retinoic acid. After a few months of taking eight pills per day, the results were dramatic. "First his tumor shrank and then…it disappeared," said Dr. Michael Hawkins, head of developmental oncology at Lombardi. While Steve Otto's experiences are not typical, they do illustrate the power of antioxidants, when the right substance is used. Steve Otto summed it up: "This has been the best adventure of my life. Look at me. I'm not supposed to be here."

By placing Accutane directly in cervical caps, doctors were also able to get an 80 percent response rate in moderate cases of cervical dysplasia. Beta-carotene and folic acid also benefit this condition.

Promyelocytic Leukemia

The vitamin A derivative called ATRA (all-trans-retinoic acid) is now a standard treatment for acute promyelocytic leukemia (APL). ATRA can quite predictably cause the disappearance of these cancers, although it is difficult to maintain the remissions. A decline in high blood levels of ATRA begins as early as three days after administration, since the body works hard to get rid of excess vitamin A. (342).

Kaposi's sarcoma

ATRA is also a standard treatment for Kaposi's sarcoma, a skin cancer that is most commonly associated with AIDS. In a clinical trial in France, 19 patients were evaluated: there were partial responses in eight people (42 percent), a stabilization of disease in seven patients (37 percent), and progression of the disease in four patients (21 percent).

A gradual flattening and lightening of the skin lesions was observed in people who responded to at least two months of treatment with ATRA. The average length of response to the drug was 332 days and the toxicity was relatively mild. (383)

Vitamin A and Bladder Cancer

Since the 1970s there has been strong evidence of a protective effect of vitamin A on bladder cancer. In 1995, a randomized clinical trial was carried out at the University of Bern, Switzerland, with a vitamin A analog called etretinate. The time between recurrences averaged 12.7 months in the placebo group but was extended to 20.3 months in the etretinate group. Consequently, the number of surgical operations that patients had to submit to was reduced in half in the etretinate group from an average of 2.1 to less than 1 per year. (424)

Fenretinide and Breast Cancer

In late 1999, Italian scientists reported that a vitamin A analog, Fenretinide, had no effect on the incidence of second breast malignancies in women who had had breast cancer. A possible benefit was seen in premenopausal women, but further studies were called for. (459a)

Vitamin A and Chemotherapy

We have spoken of oncologists' fears that vitamin A and other anitoxidants might interfere with chemotherapy. This question has been intensively investigated in the course of attempts to counteract the extreme toxicity of Adriamycin (doxorubicin). Adriamycin is an anthracycline, an anticancer drug whose action depends in part on the generation of free radicals. Other drugs in this class include daunorubicin, epirubicin, and idarubicin. Each can cause both acute and delayed toxicity, most devastatingly to the heart muscle.

Some oncologists claim that Adriamycin is "vulnerable to interaction with antioxidants." Therefore, they say, doctors should "avoid concurrent administration" of the two classes of substances. (222) **However, neither vitamin A nor any other antioxidant interferes with Adriamycin.** In fact, when laboratory animals were pretreated with vitamin A, this not only substantially reduced the damage to their heart lipids (fats) and proteins, but increased their survival. (445)

In the test tube, "an enhanced cell death was observed when the cell colony was exposed to both compounds," said Italian scientists. **"These data strongly encourage a new therapeutic approach with safe doses of vitamin A as an adjuvant in cancer chemotherapy."** (69)

Here are some other examples of how vitamin A interacts with chemotherapy in a positive way:

- A vitamin A analog, isotretinoin, had "additive anti-leukemic effects" when combined with the standard drugs vincristine or daunorubicin. There was no sign of interference. (352)
- In Rome, scientists used retinoids with the drugs beta-interferon and tamoxifen as a treatment for metastatic breast cancer. The median survival in such patients was 28 months, with 25 percent of patients alive after nine years. Again, there was no suggestion of interference between the retinoids and the other agents. (371)
- In Japan, scientists studied a combination of vitamin A with standard chemotherapy drugs. The vitamin considerably enhanced the antitumor effects of 5-FU, methotrexate, ACNU, 6-MP, and cisplatin. (306)

Clinical Trials

These laboratory studies were later extended to hundreds of human patients. As expected, the activity of 5-FU was increased by the addition of vitamin A. In fact, in Japan this combination became known as the "FAR" protocol, which stands for 5-FU, vitamin A, and radiation. It is used for cancers of the larynx, pharynx, and esophagus. Japanese doctors note a **"highly effective synergism"** (mutually enhancing activity) when they use these agents in combination. (211, 212)

In 1985, Dr. Lucien Israel reported on a group of 100 patients with metastatic breast cancer who were treated by chemotherapy as well as huge daily doses of 350,000 to 500,000 IU of vitamin A. (This should only be done under a physician's care, as high doses of vitamin A can be toxic.) Dr. Israel reported a **"significant increase in the complete response rate"** over what is generally obtainable with chemotherapy alone. The response rates, duration of response, and projected survival were all significantly increased. (180)

To summarize: Vitamin A and its derivatives have an important role in cancer prevention and treatment. I have found no evidence that this class of antioxidants interferes with any anticancer drug. On the contrary, there is an impressive body of evidence that it protects against the side effects of toxic therapies while increasing their effectiveness.

I recommend 10,000 to 20,000 International Units (IU) per day of vitamin A for all people trying to prevent cancer. There are signs that larger amounts are beneficial for cancer patients, but these should only be taken under the supervision of a physician.

6. Beta-Carotene

Carotenoids are natural plant pigments that provide the reds, oranges, yellows and other brilliant colors in nature's palette. Carotenoids are what make fruits and vegetables attractive to the eye. For decades, they were dismissed as mere food colorants, but today we have come to understand that eating them is vitally important to our health.

There are about 600 carotenoids in nature, of which about 20 have been identified in common foods. Of these, six appear most important:

Carotenoid	*Food Sources*
Beta-carotene	carrots, broccoli, cantaloupe, spinach, kale
Lutein	corn, green leafy vegetables, egg yolk
Lycopene	tomatoes, watermelon
Zeaxanthin	corn, oranges, egg yolk, green vegetables, peppers
Alpha-carotene	carrots, pumpkins
Cryptoxanthin	papayas, peaches, tangerines, oranges

People who eat foods rich in carotenoids are less likely to develop degenerative diseases and cancer than those who get few of these powerful food factors. In this chapter we shall focus on beta-carotene, and in the following chapter on the other carotenoids. Let us glance at some of the studies:

Breast

Two studies show that women with breast cancer have lower levels of beta-carotene in their blood, and a lower intake of beta-carotene in their food. (309, 354)

Head and Neck

Increased intake of fruits and vegetables is associated with a reduced risk of head-and-neck cancers. (146) In addition, there was a decrease in second primary tumors when people took more beta-carotene. (24)

Uterine

Beta-carotene blood levels are lower in women with cervical cancer than in normal controls. (339) Serum levels of total carotenoids, as well as two specific carotenoids (cryptoxanthin and alpha-carotene) were lower in people with cancer. (27) Increased dietary beta-carotene intake is also associated with a decreased risk of endometrial cancer. (310)

Lung

People with a high intake of fruits and vegetables containing beta-carotene have lower rates of lung cancer. (329) In fact, men with the lowest blood levels of beta-carotene have a 3.4 times greater risk of lung cancer than men with the highest scores. (319) There are nearly 20 studies showing an inverse relationship between dietary carotenoids and lung cancer.

In fact, since the strongest correlation was between high beta-carotene and low lung cancer rates, this is where most subsequent research efforts were focused. The results of those big trials were quite astonishing...but not in the expected way.

Beta-Carotene and Lung Cancer Prevention

Let us now focus on the famous beta-carotene and lung cancer studies. Because of beta-carotene's close association with vitamin A, it became the subject of intense scrutiny, with hundreds of scientific papers. For example, a big Westinghouse Electric study showed that men who smoked but had high levels of beta-carotene in their diet had a lower risk of lung cancer than other smokers. In fact, smokers with the highest beta-carotene intake had rates of lung cancer similar to nonsmokers!

In the 1980s, there were two major studies in which participants were given synthetic beta-carotene to see if it would prevent lung cancer. I need to tell this story in some detail, since it comes up every time the topic of antioxidants and cancer is raised.

The Finnish Alpha Tocopherol Beta Carotene (ATBC) trial enrolled 30,000 middle-aged male smokers between 1985 and 1993. These men were randomized to receive daily supplements (of either vitamin E or beta-carotene) or placebo for five to eight years. (15) After that time, the results were analyzed. Taking 50 milligrams per day of vitamin E had no effect on the lung cancer incidence among these smokers. That was disappointing enough. But synthetic beta-carotene supplements were associated with a small, but non-significant, *increase* in their death rate. Scientists thought this might have been a statistical fluke. (4)

CARET

Next came CARET, the Carotene and Retinol Efficacy Trial. This was designed by the U.S. National Cancer Institute (NCI) as one of its major trials. The purpose was to find out if 30 milligrams per day of synthetic beta-carotene and 25,000 IU of vitamin A could reduce the incidence of lung cancer in high-risk populations. The subjects were either smokers or people known to have been exposed to asbestos, which can cause a kind of lung cancer.

CARET began in 1985 with full-scale recruitment starting in 1989. The goal was 18,000 participants, about a fourth of whom were asbestos-exposed men, while the rest were either former or present smokers. Half the participants were given synthetic beta-carotene and vitamin A. The other half were given placebos.

On January 18, 1996, NCI announced that the study was being canceled eighteen months early. A statistical check had shown that one of the two groups was experiencing a higher rate of cancer. To prevent half of the participants from possibly being harmed, the secret code of the "blinded" study was broken. It turned out that the higher cancer rate was in the beta-carotene and vitamin A group: 28 percent more lung cancers and 17 percent more deaths from all causes in the vitamin-treated group.

Needless to say, these results were surprising and disappointing. They put a damper on the belief that one or two nutrients could be a "magic bullet" for cancer.

We are still suffering from the after effects of these studies. In fact, every attempt to rekindle interest in antioxidants is invariably met with, "What about CARET?" In fact, many scientists now advise the public not to take beta-carotene supplements. (329)

Beta-Carotene and Pancreatic Cancer

Not all the conclusions from the Finnish study were negative. Further analysis showed that beta-carotene actually decreased the incidence and mortality from pancreatic cancer. Incidence was 25 percent lower in men receiving beta-carotene supplements compared to those who did not receive it, and their death rate was 19 percent lower. (370) This received almost no publicity, compared to the uproar that followed the negative findings.

Meaning of the Negative Studies

We know from many other studies that the presence of vitamin A and beta-carotene in the diet is associated with lower rates of cancer and other diseases. At the same time, *synthetic* beta-carotene supplements either do nothing or increase the death rate of smokers. How can we resolve this paradox? The meaning of the CARET and Finnish studies is still being debated. There are several possible explanations of these negative findings.

The Single Carotenoid Issue

Beta-carotene is one of many dietary carotenoids. They form a close-knit network, what Robert Atkins, M.D. calls a "nutritional collective." (19) Giving one alone may upset the natural balance that occurs when lots of fruits and vegetables are taken as food. For instance, lutein and beta-carotene inhibit each others' absorption into the bloodstream. It is possible that each one keeps the other from "going overboard" in its biological effects. (453)

"Their therapeutic worth may be only as good as the weakest link in the chain," says Dr. Atkins, "and an overload of one could compromise the work of the others." He points out that the *synthetic* form lowers the blood's concentrations of such carotenes as lycopene, which have their own health-promoting properties. (454) Thus, ironically, giving too much of one carotenoid decreases the others, and may paradoxically lower one's resistance to cancer.

The Synthetic Carotene Issue

The distinction between natural and synthetic supplements is controversial, but scientists have shown there can be important differences between the two. As noted, CARET participants were given a *synthetic* form of beta-carotene. This may have affected the results.

In 1989, Israeli researchers showed that *natural* beta-carotene contains a balanced mixture of chemicals. There is also a tenfold higher accumulation of natural beta-carotene in the livers of lab animals than of synthetic beta-carotene. In prophetic words, they wrote, "Attention should be paid to the different sources of beta-carotene when testing their efficacy...such as in their possible role in the prevention of some types of cancer." (29) Scientists did not pay attention to this advice.

Another study at the University of Illinois concluded that the difference forms of beta-carotene could affect the amount actually absorbed by test animals. (470) **A 1995 paper showed that natural beta-carotene could reverse cancerous changes in stomach cancer cells, while synthetic beta-carotene could not.** (478)

The composition of natural and synthetic beta-carotene is so different that they are really different substances. A Chinese study showed that natural beta-carotene contains 40 percent of the all-trans form of the vitamin and 38 percent of the 9-cis form. By contrast, synthetic beta-carotene is overwhelming (97 percent) "all-trans," while the "9-cis" isomer cannot be detected at all. (476)

Probably because of this, synthetic beta-carotene is much less effective at protecting cells from the genetic damage that causes cancer. Chinese researchers concluded that synthetic beta-carotene could actually be harmful to the genes while natural beta-carotene "could be of practical value in tumor prevention and supplementary treatment." (476) In these experiments, natural and synthetic beta-carotenes had entirely opposite effects on tumor formation.

The 'Walking Time-Bomb' Issue

Lester Packer, Ph.D., of the University of California, Berkeley, has called CARET participants "walking time bombs." They had all been heavily exposed to asbestos, tobacco and/or alcohol. "It may simply have been too late to make a difference for this group," he says.

Beta-carotene, he remarks, mainly breaks down into vitamin A, but also into some "abnormal compounds" in tiny concentrations. These are harmless to most people, but when combined with cigarette smoke (itself the source of 200 chemicals) they may have promoted the growth of malignant cells. He concludes that "if you smoke and/or have been exposed to asbestos, you should not take supplementary beta-carotene." (335) Others would limit this restriction to the synthetic form alone.

Almost everyone agrees that natural beta-carotene in food is protective against cancer. Thus, it is still an excellent idea for smokers and others to eat lots of colorful fruits and vegetables on a regular basis. If you do take a carotene supplement, make sure that it is (a) of natural origin and (b) contains a mixture of carotenoids.

Despite CARET, there have been some more recent studies showing benefits even from beta-carotene taken as a single agent. Thus, Dr. Michelle S. Santos of the USDA Human Nutrition Center on Aging at Tufts University, Boston, had reported that long-term supplementation with beta-carotene daily for older men results in the kind of immune system activity normally seen in men 20 years younger. This was particularly true of natural killer (NK) cells. (386) In addition, "the effects of dietary antioxidants are mainly demonstrated in connection with age-associated diseases in which oxidative stress appears to be intimately involved." (279)

Beta-carotene is to get a second chance in France. A huge study called "Suvimax" has been launched. Suvimax is an acronym for "Supplementation en Vitamines et Mineraux Antioxydants." This is large and scientifically rigorous study whose main objective is to evaluate a combination of antioxidant vitamins and minerals at nutritional (not high-dose) levels. Almost 13,000 volunteers of both sexes have been signed up in France, and the study will take at least eight years. Studying cancer and heart disease rates are the main points of the project. (112)

Beta-Carotene and Chemotherapy

Does beta-carotene interfere with radiation and chemotherapy, as some oncologists fear?

No, it does not. A 1996 laboratory study showed that beta-carotene reduced the heart damage of the drug Adriamycin. (256) In a study at the Dana-Farber Cancer Institute in Boston, beta-carotene did not interfere with Adriamycin's cell-killing ability. Beta-carotene combined with Adriamycin (as well as other conventional anticancer drugs) showed an increased destruction of tumor cells and a greater delay in the growth of tumors than when these drugs were used alone. (444)

Beta-Carotene and Cisplatin

A study at Harvard University showed that beta-carotene reduced the toxicity of the standard drug cisplatin. Together with vitamin E, it increased the level of certain detoxification enzymes, a sign that toxicity could be reduced. (397)

Beta-Carotene and Melphalan, BCNU, Etoposide

The combination of beta-carotene with the toxic drug melphalan (L-PAM) was particularly impressive. (397) In general, beta-carotene and/or the vitamin A analog, 13-cis retinoic acid, works well with L-PAM, BCNU, and etoposide, among other toxic agents. (444)

To summarize: Beta-carotene is a powerful and necessary antioxidant, which is available in many foods, as well as in natural supplement forms. Unlike vitamin A, beta-carotene is very safe, even in high doses. I have found no studies showing that beta-carotene interferes with the actions of radiation or chemotherapy. Most studies report that it helps decrease the side effects of these treatments.

7. *Other Carotenoids*

Until recently, the controversy over beta-carotene obscured exciting developments using the lesser-known carotenoids against cancer. Most experiments have been done with them collectively, and in fact they are best studied (and taken) as a complex.

Lutein and Zeaxanthin

Lutein helps give apricots, oranges, peaches, and summer squashes their attractive yellow to light-orange color. The richest source is green leafy vegetables such as kale, spinach, and collard greens. These do not appear yellow because lutein pigments are masked by the dominant green chlorophyll pigment. The name *zeaxanthin* refers to the yellow color of corn. Together, these two carotenoids help protect various delicate tissues from free radical damage. Lutein even beats beta-carotene at protecting fats inside eye cells from such damage.

Lutein and Cancer

"Lutein and lycopene possess exceptionally high antioxidant capacity compared to other carotenoids and may be useful in preventing cancer," said Dr. Fred Khachik, a chemist with the U.S. Department of Agriculture. **Lutein promotes healthy immunity and decreases the growth of cancer.** There are already over 250 scientific papers referring to lutein's potential as an anticancer agent. And lutein is five times more readily available from vegetables than beta-carotene. (453)

Lutein has many beneficial effects in experimental animals. It increases the time until the tumor appears, suppresses the growth of breast tumors, and also enhances the growth of normal white blood cells. (340) What was particularly exciting was that very low amounts of lutein, comprising no more than two-thousands of the overall diet by weight, "can efficiently decrease mammary [breast] tumor development and growth in mice." (341)

At Japan's National Cancer Center Research Institute in Tokyo, scientists showed that lutein protects against the formation of colon cancer, as measured by the number of pre-cancers per mouse. (203, 308)

Alpha-Carotene

Alpha-carotene is a little known cousin of beta-carotene. Japanese scientists have shown that alpha-carotene is better than its more famous relative at suppressing cancer formation in experimental animals. (317) This could have practical implications. A little noted 1999 study from the University of California, San Diego, showed that **the best way to get alpha-carotene and lutein into one's diet is through the consumption of fresh vegetable juices.** (270) Juicing is a part of many unconventional cancer treatment programs.

Lycopene

Lycopene is a natural carotenoid, which is responsible for the bright red color of tomatoes and a number of other foods.

Lycopene Content of Commonly Eaten Foods

Food	*Portion*	*Milligrams Lycopene*
Spaghetti sauce	five ounces	21
Processed vegetable juice	one glass	17
Fresh, red tomatoes	five ounces	14
Watermelon	ten ounces	11
Pizza sauce	per one slice	10
Canned tomato paste	one ounce	9
Ketchup	one tablespoon	3

"The data strongly suggests that tomato products should be a component of a healthy dietary pattern that includes at least five servings of fruits and vegetables per day," says Dr. Steven K. Clinton of the Dana-Farber Cancer Institute, Boston.

"The beneficial effects of tomato products have been clearly demonstrated," according to Dr. John Weisburger of the American Health Foundation in Valhalla, New York.

Much of the excitement over lycopene has to do with its ability to reduce the risk of heart disease by preventing the oxidation of low density lipoproteins (LDL). A report in the journal *Lipids* showed that daily consumption of tomato products (providing at least 40 milligrams of lycopene) could substantially reduce the oxidation of LDL, thus lowering heart disease rates. (1)

Lycopene and Cancer

When lycopene is cultured with human endometrial, breast, and lung cancer cells, it is four times stronger than alpha-carotene, and ten times stronger than beta-carotene at inhibiting tumor growth.

Israeli scientists theorize that lycopene suppresses an insulin-like growth factor that stimulates tumors. This may "open new avenues for research on the role of lycopene in the regulation of endometrial cancer and other tumors," they wrote. (232)

Pharmacologists in Milan, Italy, have also shown that high intake of tomatoes is associated with a:

- 35 percent reduction in cancer of the oral cavity, pharynx and esophagus;
- 57 percent reduction in cancer of the stomach;
- 58 percent reduction in cancer of the rectum; and
- 61 percent reduction in cancer of the colon.

In fact, they believe that much of the health benefits of the Mediterranean diet can be attributed to the extensive consumption of tomatoes and tomato products. (221)

Lycopene and Prostate Cancer

Recently, most attention has focused on the relationship of lycopene to prostate cancer. According to Edward Giovannucci, M.D., of the Harvard School of Public Health, Boston, tomato products contribute to a reduction in the chances of men getting prostate cancer. (134)

Of 46 foods tested, four were associated with lower prostate cancer risk and three of these were major sources of lycopene: tomato sauce, fresh tomatoes and pizza. (The fourth was strawberries, rich in other antioxidants.) Men who ate ten servings per week of tomato products had one-third less risk of prostate cancer than those who consumed a mere 1.5 servings per week. And they had only half the risk of having advanced stages of the disease. (134, 135)

Digestive Tract

People who eat pizza and other tomato-rich foods are also less likely to get cancer of the stomach or digestive tract. (122, 483)

Prostate Cancer

A very promising 1999 report showed that supplements of lycopene slow the growth of prostate cancer. Dr. Omar Kucuk of the Barbara Ann Karmanos Cancer Institute in Detroit found that **lycopene supplements slowed prostate cancer in men diagnosed with the disease.** Thirty men, who had prostate cancer and were waiting to have surgery, were given a tomato concentrate pill daily. The other half received placebos. Then all the mens' tumors were examined after they had surgery.

"The men who took lycopene had lower PSA levels in their tumors," said Dr. Kucuk. The tumors of the men who took lycopene were also smaller when they finally had surgery. **"This shows that lycopene may not only be possibly preventive for prostate cancer but may possibly in the future play a role in treatment,"** Kucuk told a news conference.

To summarize: One should try to consume 40 milligrams of lycopene per day. You can get almost this much by drinking two glasses of tomato juice (or V8). If you do not like tomatoes, or cannot get this amount though your daily diet, as per the above chart, you could take a lycopene supplement.

8. Vitamin C

Vitamin C, or ascorbic acid, is the cornerstone of any antioxidant program. It is an extraordinary molecule that performs hundreds of essential functions. In a way, vitamin C defines us as a species, since (along with guinea pigs, fruit-eating bats, and the red-vented bulbul bird) we primates are the only animals who must forage for our daily supply, while the rest of the animals make it themselves.

If we don't get any vitamin C, we come down with scurvy. This disease was particularly common on long sea voyages, and more than a million sailors died of it during the eighteenth and nineteenth centuries. The great explorers, like Vasco da Gama and Magellan, lost half their crews to scurvy, and that was not considered unusual.

Vitamin C was first isolated (from Hungarian red peppers) by my mentor, Albert Szent-Györgyi. It was a brilliant discovery for which he won the 1937 Nobel Prize. Vitamin C is now among the most thoroughly researched substances in the world, the subject of over 20,000 scientific articles.

Preventing and curing scurvy turned out to be just the first of vitamin C's many triumphs. "C" is crucial for the production of antibodies and for immune power in general. It is central to wound healing and to recovery from surgery—cancer patients take note!

In a randomized clinical trial in Russia, vitamin C, along with vitamins A and E were given to prevent postoperative complications in 197 people with stomach cancer. The complication rate dropped dramatically from 30.9 to 1.9 percent. (428)

In fact, vitamin C helps cement the body together by forming a fibrous connective tissue called collagen. It is also a natural antihistamine, which reduces the symptoms of allergy and asthma. It also prevents cataracts, aids in the formation of liver bile, helps to detoxify alcohol and other substances—the list goes on.

Vitamin C also lessens the duration and severity of colds. It blocks the activation of viral genes. And it plays a role—possibly a crucial one—in the prevention and treatment of cardiovascular disease.

Vitamin C and Cancer

Given its amazing versatility, is it any wonder that Dr. Linus Pauling and his many followers, believed that this super-vitamin could also combat cancer? We shall leave the treatment claims for last. If we look at the question of prevention, however, **there is little doubt that a diet high in vitamin C reduces the risk of cancer substantially.** Its mode of action is multiple. It protects the genetic material from free radical damage, strengthens the immune system, and increases resistance to harmful chemicals. Another recently discovered function is to boost the other antioxidants, particularly vitamin E. (335)

Evidence from the Field

Scientists who study varying rates of cancer among different populations have repeatedly shown that people with a low consumption of citrus fruits and other vitamin C-containing foods have higher rates of stomach cancer. (37,148,169,210,276) Some of these studies were conducted on the shores of the Caspian Sea in Iran and northeastern Turkey, where the local population has unusually high rates of cancer of the esophagus. It was discovered that in this region, esophageal cancer was associated with a low intake of vitamin C-rich fruits and vegetables. (81,277)

After publication of this data, reports began to come in on similar associations of low vitamin C intake with high rates of cancer.

- In Buffalo, New York, scientists found that vitamin C protected against cancer of the larynx. (143)
- In the Bronx, New York, low vitamin C consumption was associated with cervical dysplasia, a common premalignant condition of women. There was a ten-fold increase in this condition among those who had the lowest intake of vitamin C. (466)
- In Canada, vitamin C intake had the most consistent and statistically significant inverse association with breast cancer risk. Those who consumed the most vitamin C had a third less breast cancer than those who got the least. Vitamin C-rich diets resulted in a 16 to 24 percent reduction in breast cancer risk.
- In Boston, a 1999 Harvard study of over 83,000 nurses showed a strong inverse association between high vitamin C intake (from foods) and breast cancer in *premenopausal* women with a positive family history of the disease. (481) **The more vitamin C and other**

antioxidants in the diet, the less breast cancer.

- In Greece, scientists also found an association between low vitamin C intake and cancer in *postmenopausal* women. (43)

Are you surprised to learn this? These amazing findings get almost no press, while proposals for "chemoprevention" using toxic and carcinogenic synthetic drugs dominate the news. Vitamin C never had and never will have the kind of money behind it that patented pharmaceuticals do.

Vitamin C at the Breakfast Table

Vitamin C may be responsible for the sharp decline in stomach cancer, which used to be the most prevalent form of cancer in the United States. Around 1930, incidence and deaths began to fall. This decline coincided with the advent of frozen orange juice in America's diet. Vitamin C in breakfast orange juice probably blocked the formation of carcinogens (called nitrosamines) in the stomachs of people eating bacon or ham and eggs. (75, 285) The Japanese, who do not generally drink orange juice, continue to have very high rates of stomach cancer.

Inhibition of Cancer

Vitamin C can inhibit the conversion of a normal to a cancerous cell after exposure to a carcinogen. And cancer cells turn back into normal-appearing cells when you add vitamin C to the culture medium. (178, 378) Vitamin C also blocks the initiation of cancer by X rays. (477)

Vitamin C as a Cancer Treatment

The intravenous administration of vitamin C dates to the 1940s when Fred Klenner, M.D. used it to treat patients suffering from viral diseases. (206) Klenner later said, **"ascorbic acid is the safest and the most valuable substance available to the physician. Many headaches and many heartaches will be avoided with its proper use."**

The idea of intravenous, high-dose vitamin C was revived by Ewan Cameron, M.D. and Linus Pauling, Ph.D., as a treatment for advanced cancer. Cameron was a highly regarded surgeon at the Vale of Leven Hospital in West Central Scotland who worked with vitamin C and cancer patients for several decades.

Both men believed that vitamin C would be of value in protecting against the "destructive effects of malignant invasiveness" by stabilizing the body and enhancing the formation of the cellular cement called collagen.

In 1991, they reported on results in 294 advanced cancer patients who received supplemental vitamin C at some stage in their illness. These were compared with 1,532 cancer patients at the same hospital who did not receive the vitamin. The vitamin C patients had an average overall survival time of 343 days, compared with 180 days for the non-vitamin group. There was a lot of medical skepticism about these results, and Cameron and Pauling experienced enormous difficulties in getting their observation published in a scientific journal. (58)

Cameron recommended that all cancer patients be given an initial course of intravenous vitamin C followed by a maintenance oral dose, continued indefinitely thereafter.

Such statements raised the ire of the medical establishment, and two clinical trials at the Mayo Clinic, intending to test their ideas, claimed there was no benefit for patients receiving high-dose vitamin C. Pauling then claimed that the Mayo Clinic tests were fraudulent. This controversy has never been resolved.

Meanwhile, there has been some additional data that supports Pauling's point of view. A series of experiments at Wayne State University, Detroit, has shown that vitamin C inhibits the growth of cancer cells. By looking at cancer cells under the electron microscope, scientists could see signs of a regular battlefield. The cancer cells were disorganized, their internal structures altered, their membranes disrupted and they were surrounded by the body's collagen cement. (258, 259)

In animals, vitamin C was shown to protect against the formation of liver cancer by carcinogens. (200)

Health Scares

Vitamin C is the flagship of the antioxidant Armada. It therefore presents an irresistible target to the inveterate opponents of alternative medicine. Many challengers have taken a turn trying to bring down vitamin C. None has succeeded.

"Harmful effects have been mistakenly attributed to vitamin C, including hypoglycemia, rebound scurvy, infertility, mutagenesis [formation of mutations], and destruction of vitamin B12," wrote Mark Levine in the *Journal of the American Medical Association* in 1999. **"Health professionals should recognize that vitamin C does not produce these effects."** (230)

The Food and Nutrition Board of the National Academy of Sciences' Institute of Medicine concurred. They are formulating new "dietary reference intakes" for the healthy U.S. population. One of their tasks is to determine any adverse effects of high-dose vitamin C and to "define and defend" a Tolerable Upper Intake Level. An admirable task—but they finally admitted they couldn't find one! As they put it, the **"available data indicate that very high intakes of vitamin C (2-4 grams per day) are well tolerated biologically in healthy mammalian systems."** (187)

Since I do not advocate doses that high, even for cancer patients, I could leave it at that. However, in the real world you will be confronted by various anti-vitamin C myths if you pursue this topic. I would therefore like to present you with some more facts about these fallacious arguments.

Kidney Stones

Some years ago there was a big scare that high doses of vitamin C would lead to kidney stone formation. Since kidney stones are among the most painful of human afflictions, this was a serious charge. The concern was entirely theoretical: vitamin C can turn into oxalate in the body and oxalate is the basis of some kidney stones. But this association is incorrect.

Recent reports have shown that blood levels of vitamin C are not associated with an increased prevalence of kidney stones in men or women. (409) According to a South African researcher, "ingestion of large doses of ascorbic acid does not affect the principal risk factors associated with calcium oxalate kidney stone formation."(21)

In 1999, there was a report from Harvard Medical School, Boston, that looked at over 85,000 women with kidney stones. It showed conclusively that women who took high-dose vitamin C (1,500 milligrams or more per day) had no excess of kidney stones. On the other hand, taking at least 40 milligrams per day of vitamin B6 reduced kidney stone formation by one third. **"Routine restriction of vitamin C to prevent stone formation appears unwarranted,"** they concluded. One can only wonder how this erroneous story got started and has been perpetuated for decades.

Vitamin B12 Deficiency?

Another widely publicized health scare was that high-dose vitamin C could lead to vitamin B12 deficiency. This was the position of Victor Herbert, M.D. of the Veterans' Administration hospital, Bronx, New York. Dr. Herbert put forward this view in a 1974 article in the *Journal of the American Medical Association (JAMA)*. (160) However, this claim also turned out to be unsupported by subsequent research.

As early as 1976, an article in the *American Journal of Clinical Nutrition*, based on the findings of two independent laboratories, concluded "there was no deleterious effect of added ascorbic acid on the vitamin B12 content of meals." (316)

It was later reported in another *JAMA* article that the earlier association of vitamin C with diminished vitamin B12 was apparently caused by the "incomplete protection of the extracted vitamin B12 in the assay [testing] procedure." (315) Other scientists called the original reports "artifacts of the methods used" and "highly improbable." (264)

Serum levels of vitamin C were **"not associated with decreased serum vitamin B12 levels (or indicators of vitamin B12 deficiency)...."** according to a recent study of 9,250 individuals in the Second National Health and Nutrition Examination Survey, which was published by scientists at the Veterans Administration hospital in San Francisco.

In fact, higher blood levels of vitamin C were associated with a small *increase* in vitamin B12. (409)

Despite such factual refutations, one still hears the same erroneous charges about vitamin C depleting vitamin B12 at scientific meetings and in public forums. Old rumors die hard.

Pro-Oxidant?

Another health scare came from England in 1998 and was widely publicized in the *New York Times.* This study claimed that while vitamin C was an effective antioxidant at lower doses, at high doses (which were defined as 500 milligrams per day), it could cause cellular damage. Scientists tracked two indicators of oxidation damage in the genetic material of 30 healthy volunteers. One of these obscure markers showed *less*, but the other showed *more*, oxidation. (353)

It is well known that the same nutrient can function as an antioxidant or a pro-oxidant, depending on the context (398). Yet these particular findings contradict many other studies showing that vitamin C basically functions as an antioxidant in the human body. The marker in question has not been proven to be a good indicator of oxidative stress or cell damage, and the study unleashed a storm of criticism.

"I was sort of shocked this received the sort of play it did," said Dr. David Golde, physician-in-chief at Memorial Sloan-Kettering Cancer Center in New York. Dr. Golde said he believed the study was **"technically flawed...The data is all over the place...It doesn't make any sense..."**

Dr. Mark Levine, chief of molecular and clinical nutrition at the National Institutes of Health, told reporters, "How can I put this simply? I think the conclusion is **not justified by the data.**" He said the study was flawed because researchers measured the level of vitamin C in the blood but not the level of vitamin C in the cells.

Dr. Jeffrey Blumberg, chief of the antioxidant research lab in the Human Research Center at Tufts University in Boston, said that 500 milligrams is a reasonable amount to take. "This is bad science," he added.

As Professor Balz Frei of the Linus Pauling Institute at Oregon State University, said, "The value of vitamin C in lowering the risk of cancer, heart disease, and other serious health problems must be considered in its totality, not just in a focus on one single aspect of its biological effect."

What I find particularly astonishing is that later in 1998, the authors of the original study published another report on vitamin C. This showed that people who received 500 milligrams of vitamin C per day had substantial benefit from the practice!

"These results illustrate...a role for vitamin C in the regulation of DNA repair enzymes," and demonstrate an "antioxidant effect," they wrote. (82)

Did you hear about these pro-vitamin C results? Probably not, because unlike the scare stories, these positive findings and comments passed without mention in the mainstream media.

The Golde Study

David W. Golde, the aforementioned physician-in-chief of Memorial Sloan-Kettering, has published a series of technical articles on vitamin C. He has shown that some tumors accumulate high amounts of vitamin C. (2) Based on this, he raised concerns in the media about using vitamin C at the same time as chemotherapy, telling *Science News* that "vitamin C might make cancer treatment less effective" (10/2/99).

This conclusion is based on fear, not fact. High concentrations of vitamin C in experimental tumors is not proof that vitamin C is harmful to cancer patients. It is an old observation that some tumors are high in vitamin C, and nobody really knows what it is doing there. It may be a good thing.

By analogy, Dr. Golde himself has shown that HIV-infected cells also soak up vitamin C, and yet, to quote a 1997 Sloan-Kettering press release, "extremely high levels of the vitamin are more toxic to the HIV-infected cells than to healthy immune cells."

Dr. Golde's fears are a reflection of the prevailing attitude among many oncologists, who use drugs of exceptionally high toxicity, but balk at their patients' use of non-toxic nutritional supplements.

Iron Overload?

There is one area in which I think that concerns over vitamin C intake may be justified. About one in 5,000 people of Northern European descent has a hereditary disorder called hemochromatosis. Such people have a genetic mutation that results in excessive iron absorption. This is a potentially dangerous condition and there have been hints that vitamin C leads to elevated iron levels in people with this condition. (132)

For that reason, scientists at the Veterans Administration Hospital in San Francisco suggest that people with a genetic susceptibility to iron overload should moderate their intake of ascorbic acid. (409) I agree.

Proper Dose

A consensus is emerging that the minimum daily requirement of vitamin C should be more than the current RDA, which is 60 milligrams per day for most people. Dr. Balz Frei has called for an increase to 120 milligrams per day. Mark Levine, M.D., writing in the *Journal of the American Medical Association*, has called for raising the daily amount to 200 milligrams per day. (231) Doses above 400 milligrams per day, said Levine, had "no evident value." (230)

Andrew Weil, M.D., who once recommended megadoses, now suggests 250 to 500 milligrams per day, in divided doses.

This is a reasonable amount for people who are not actively fighting cancer. But cancer and its treatment place great stress on a person. It is therefore prudent for people with cancer to take more.

Animals under stress increase their production of vitamin C by two or three times. Therefore, people with cancer could take one or two grams per day, in divided doses. This is a fraction of what many people have taken for years with no ill effects.

Vitamin C and Adriamycin

Does vitamin C interfere with chemotherapy? The short answer is, No. As with other antioxidants, this question was first intensively investigated in relation to Adriamycin (doxorubicin).

It is was found that vitamin C "can protect normal cells from the damage caused by [free] radicals without interfering with the cytotoxicity of doxorubicin against tumors." (16, 17)

Many animal studies have confirmed that the combination of Adriamycin and vitamin C significantly prolonged the life of animals treated treated with both. (10, 124, 154, 215, 405, 442) In general, instead of interference, there is a **"consistent synergism" of vitamin C and Adriamycin.** (219)

Vitamin C and Cisplatin

Cisplatin is another powerful, but toxic, anticancer drug that causes chromosomal damage, mutations in bone marrow cells, and abnormalities in sperm. When vitamin C is added, the numbers of such mutations "were always significantly less than that treated with cisplatin alone." This suggested, scientists say, a "protective role of ascorbic acid against cisplatin's toxicity." (136, 362)

Vitamin C and Levodopa

Scientists at Washington State University looked at the interaction of vitamin C and an experimental drug for melanoma called levodopa methylester (LDME). In animals, vitamin C not only inhibited tumor growth but enhanced LDME's activity and increased survival. Metastases were inhibited in mice that received vitamin C. This work has been repeatedly confirmed. (47, 126, 127, 272, 348, 349, 457)

Clinical Study of Chemotherapy, Vitamin C and Vitamin K3

A series of experiments at the Catholic University of Louvain, Belgium, showed a synergy (additive effect) between vitamin C and vitamin K3 and six different forms of chemotherapy. Adding the vitamins increased the effect of all of the drugs, especially when the vitamins were injected just before chemotherapy.

But this additive effect did not increase the toxicity either to the animals in general or to any specific organ. (439) Vitamins C and K3 worked together very well.

When cancer cells become resistant to chemotherapy, vitamins can help restore their sensitivity. The Belgian doctors suggested that adding these vitamins "into classical protocols of human cancer treatment would be without any supplementary risk." (88, 440)

Extravasation?

Devastating leaks can occur whenever highly toxic and corrosive drugs like Adriamycin are given intravenously. The drugs can leak out of the intravenous tubes and traumatize the patient (or even the nurse), causing skin ulceration and "significant morbidity."

Such accidents are called extravasation. Scientists in Oregon have found a potential solution. If Adriamycin is delivered in a solution of vitamin C, it lowers the rate of skin ulcers from 87 to 27 percent in an experimental animal system. (149)

Vitamin C and Polyposis of the Colon

Several randomized clinical trials have been performed using vitamin C as a treatment for polyposis of the colon. Over a two-year period, 49 patients were tested. Early results were positive. A follow-up study found a 14 percent reduction. (271) An Italian trial showed the greatest benefit: in 209 patients, the percentages of recurrence were about one-seventh in the vitamin C group. However, the largest American study (which used vitamins A, C and E) found no benefit. (144) At the moment, there is no consensus that vitamin C helps prevent polyposis.

Prasad Experiments

More recently, Dr. Kedar Prasad, of the University of Colorado, published extensive laboratory experiments on the effects of vitamin C alone, as well as in combination with various anticancer agents. (357)

Combinations of Vitamin C and Conventional Agents

Agent Used	Decrease in Cancer Growth
Vitamin C	-5.0%*
5-FU	38.0%
5-FU + vitamin C	95.5%
X rays	72.0%
X rays + vitamin C	98.2%
Bleomycin	73.0%
Bleomycin + vitamin C	92.0%

*statistically non-significant increase

Interference?

In the late 1970s, Dr. Prasad noticed that sodium ascorbate (a form of vitamin C) had varying effects on different chemotherapy drugs. Using neuroblastoma cells, he found that vitamin C added to the cancer-killing effects of many well known anticancer agents such as dacarbazine, 5-FU, bleomycin, tamoxifen, as well as X rays. A mixture of vitamin C, beta-carotene and vitamin E showed even more benefit. (359, 360)

It is ironic that one of the few negative tests on the interaction of vitamin C and chemotherapy came from Dr. Prasad, who now strongly advocates its concurrent use during chemotherapy (357). Prasad found that vitamin C *reduced* the cell-killing effects of the drugs methotrexate and DTIC in neuroblastoma cells. (360). However, he later showed that when vitamin C was joined with other antioxidants it actually *enhanced* the effect of DTIC on malignant melanoma cells. (359) As Dr. Prasad said, this showed that **"the use of single vitamins in the treatment of human cancer has no biological rationale."**

Vitamin C and Radiation

Does vitamin C interfere with radiation therapy? Dr. Prasad, a radiation researcher, showed that X rays alone killed 72 percent of the cancer cells, but **when vitamin C was added, together they killed 98.2 percent.** Similar results were seen in Belgium, where scientists noted an increase in the effectiveness of X rays, without any additional harm for the patients. (439)

A similar synergy between vitamins and radiation was demonstrated at the Massachusetts General Hospital in Boston. Writing in the *Journal of the National Cancer Institute*, scientists reported that normal tissues were protected from the harmful effects of radiation by vitamin C. (325) Vitamin C significantly increased the dose of radiation that could cause fatalities in animals. High doses of injected vitamin C were not toxic to normal cells, nor did they interfere with the cancer-controlling effects of radiation. (326)

However, there might be exceptional circumstances in which one should not take vitamin C supplements. This includes people with the hereditary disease hemochromatosis, as well as possibly some patients receiving methotrexate and DTIC.

Looking over the whole twenty-five-year controversy, Lester Packer has concluded, **"The naysayers turned out to be wrong. Their admonitions did not stop millions of people from taking megadoses of vitamin C, with few ill effects."** (335)

Kedar Prasad, Ph.D. is that rare scientist who also communicates with patients through popular writings. In addition to his professional books on radiation and antioxidants, he has written an excellent practical guide for the public, *Vitamins in Cancer Prevention and Treatment.*

In a 1999 article, Dr. Prasad challenged his colleagues to recognize high-dose multiple antioxidants as "essential ingredients in improving the efficacy of standard cancer therapy." (357) The *New York Times* noted that "Prasad and colleagues found that high doses of multiple antioxidants can not only protect normal cells during cancer treatment, but can also help fight back tumors. Together with diet and lifestyle changes, antioxidants may improve standard cancer therapy."

To summarize: **The data overwhelmingly supports an anticancer role for vitamin C, especially when it is given with radiation or chemotherapy.** There is almost no evidence for any interference. The proper dosage depends on one's circumstances. At a minimum, I suggest that you get at least 250 milligrams of vitamin C per day, in divided doses. 500 milligrams per day would be even better. Those actively fighting cancer should take between 1,000 and 2,000 milligrams per day, in divided doses.

9. Vitamin E

Vitamin E is a collective term for the most important group of fat soluble antioxidants. The cooking oil on your shelf may have vitamin E added to prevent spoilage through oxidation. In the same way, when you take vitamin E, it prevents the fatty portion of your cells from oxidizing. Oxidization means the formation of free radicals, which puts us at an increased risk of disease. Vitamin E is the mainstay of our defenses against oxidative damage to our fats.

Vitamin E's existence was theorized by two California scientists, Herbert Evans and Katherine Bishop, in 1922. They observed that laboratory rats on standard chow spontaneously aborted their pups unless they also got green lettuce to eat. The Berkeley scientists postulated the existence of some vitamin-like substance in lettuce that made normal term pregnancies possible.

Over a decade later, in 1936, this substance was finally isolated from wheat germ oil and given the name tocopherol, from the Greek words for childbirth (*tokos*) and to carry (*pherein*).

Vitamin E is found in foods, particularly raw vegetable oils, nuts and nut butters, rice bran oil and, in small quantities, green leafy vegetables.

Some writers seized on an alleged sexual connection and touted vitamin E as a restorer of youth and sexual potency. Such sensationalism further discouraged scientists from investigating this vitamin's potential. For many years, vitamin E was a popular, but not a medical, sensation.

But vitamin E's function in the body remained obscure. An extreme deficiency could cause muscle weakness and wasting. Food scientists realized that it was an antioxidant and could prevent oxidative damage. But until the free radical theory became accepted this hardly seemed relevant to human beings, since it was not yet known that fats could be oxidized inside the body.

Starting in the 1930s, two Canadian cardiologists, Wilfred and Evan Shute, began treating their heart patients with vitamin E supplements. They claimed success and their approach became a *cause celebre* of the late 1950s. They published a number of books, including their bestseller, *Vitamin E for Healthy and Ailing Hearts.*

They reported treating over 30,000 patients, with very positive results. Millions of people began taking vitamin E. Some scientists have noted the persistent decline in coronary artery disease over the past two decades and the possible contribution of antioxidants such as vitamin E to this improvement in public health. (279, 280)

At the time, the medical establishment dismissed the Shute's work as unfounded. "The notion that a simple vitamin pill could have a profound effect on the health and well-being of patients was considered absurd," wrote Lester Packer. "Back then, **preventive medicine wasn't even given lip service,** much less practiced."(335)

One problem was that no one knew how vitamin E functioned in the body. In 1954, Al Tappel of the University of California, Davis, proved that vitamin E worked in the same way inside the body as it did on the outside, by preventing fats and oils from turning rancid: it protected our body fats from what was called "lipid peroxidation."

In 1966, Dr. Raymond Shamberger of the Cleveland Clinic published the first article on the possible use of antioxidants such as vitamin E to protect against the formation of cancer. (402) Between 1966 until 1980, there were only seven articles on the topic—just one every two years. Vitamin E was derided as "a treatment in search of a disease." In the 1970s, a few non-conventional practitioners began using vitamin E (along with A and C) to "ACE the cancer," but were generally dismissed as cranks.

In the last few years, however, vitamin E has become respectable. As Dr. Kenneth Pienta of the University of Michigan wrote in 1999, "Vitamin E is one of the most researched compounds in medicine." (302) There are now 15,000 medical articles on vitamin E, and about 1,500 relate to cancer. The number of lay publications is incalculable: an Internet search turned up 55,000 items.

Already, about half of all adult Americans (including cardiologists) are taking vitamin E supplements. While orthodox oncology has not yet embraced vitamin E as a treatment, there is widespread acceptance of the idea that eating vitamin E-containing foods is associated with lower cancer rates. Prominent scientists have called for large-scale clinical trials of vitamin E as a treatment for cancer, and perhaps we shall see such tests in our lifetime.

Regulation of p53

Vitamin E, along with other antioxidants, can have a profound impact, down to the level of the genes. In 1999, a study of head-and-neck cancer patients was presented at the American Association for Cancer Research meeting. Scientists at Georgetown and other universities showed that **"regular use of any vitamin supplement corresponded to significant-**

ly reduced risk of p53 mutation." The use of vitamins A, C, and E in particular led to a four-fold reduction in p53 mutations. (50)

P53 is the most important tumor suppressor gene, which normally acts as a brake on cancerous changes in a cell. When p53 goes bad (mutates), the cell itself is launched on the path of malignancy. Signs of mutated p53 genes are found in about half of all cancers and p53 mutations are generally a sign of aggressive tumors.

The same scientists also looked at the influence of vitamins on the p53 status of smokers. Among those who had smoked for less than 29 years, **"vitamin use profoundly reduced the risk of p53 mutation."** But among those who had smoked more than 29 years, vitamin use did not significantly reduce such mutations. (50) The implications of this are profound. We think of genetic mutations as predetermined or unchangeable. Yet in this study, the genetic expression of cells was altered for the better by the addition of a few antioxidants.

Other studies confirm the power of vitamin E against cancer:

- Giving patients vitamin E for 24 weeks led to a 46 percent reduction in premalignant changes in the mouth (clinical leukoplakia). (31)
- Vitamin E combined with fish oil helps the immune systems of cancer patients. Sixty patients with a variety of advanced solid tumors were given either this mixture or a placebo. The treatment balanced the immune system and prolonged survival time of the treated patients. (138)
- Scientists in Bern, Switzerland, found that vitamin E inhibits the activity of a substance that stimulates tumor growth. **Older people who took vitamin E supplements daily were 41 percent less likely to die of cancer, and 40 percent less likely to die of heart disease, than people who did not take vitamin E.** (45)
- Another Swiss study examined almost 3,000 men over several decades. It was found that low vitamin E levels, especially in smokers, was related to an increased risk of prostate cancer. (103)
- Vitamin E controls and enhances the entire immune system. In a study at Tufts University, Boston, vitamin E significantly increased immune cell activity. Study participants reported a 30 percent lower incidence of infections than people who did not take vitamin E. (280)
- Researchers have found that the immune system relies on accurate cell-to-cell communication and any damage to this signaling system results in impaired immunity. Adequate amounts of antioxidants are absolutely necessary to prevent damage to the immune cells. Some British scientists have concluded that one needs an adequate intake of antioxidants

from an early age to prevent the development of degenerative diseases. (94)

- In late 1999, NCI scientists found that a diet rich in vitamin E can lower the risk of lung cancer among smokers by about 20 percent. The benefits were most dramatic among men under age 60 and among light smokers who had used cigarettes for less than 40 years. The reduction in lung cancer risk among these people was from 40 percent to 50 percent. (474)

What Form of Vitamin E?

Many of us pop a multivitamin or even a vitamin E pill and think we have taken care of our needs. We rarely look closely at the fine print on the label that tells us what kind of vitamin E we are getting.

There are eight forms of vitamin E. Four are tocopherols, and are named for the first four letters of the Greek alphabet. The best known is alpha-tocopherol. It has the greatest amount of vitamin E activity. However, the seven others also contribute.

Because early research focused on alpha-tocopherol, it crowded out research on the others. Some forms of vitamin E were even rejected as "junk." There have been 13,000 scientific articles on alpha-tocopherol, but only around 150 on delta-tocopherol. However, the lesser known tocopherols also have important roles to play in cancer prevention. Michigan scientists discovered that it was gamma-tocopherol, not alpha, that had the greatest anticancer activity against prostate cancer cells. (302) When you take a vitamin E supplement you should try to get all the tocopherols.

How Much Vitamin E is Enough?

Since vitamin E accumulates in fat, it is possible to take too much. The proper amount ranges from 200 to 1,200 International Units (IU), depending on the person's needs. People who are trying to prevent cancer only need 400 IU per day. People who are actively fighting cancer need 400 to 800 IU. The highest dose is for those undergoing radiation or chemotherapy, but one should not go any higher than 1,200 IU.

Few people in industrialized countries suffer from outright vitamin E deficiencies, because a small amount of the vitamin is added to many foods. But at the same time it has been processed out of many of the foods that formerly contained it. Even in a wealthy country like the U.S., people on average get only 8 IUs per day, which is half of the already minuscule RDA.

In 1999, the *Berkeley Wellness Letter* recommended that its readers take

200 to 800 IU of vitamin E, depending on the person. This was a significant recognition by a conservative medical newsletter that vitamin E plays many crucial roles in the body, and that our needs can only be met through supplementation.

Vitamin E and Chemotherapy

Does vitamin E interfere with radiation or chemotherapy? Once again, the short answer is, No. Vitamin E works well with toxic agents, reduces their side effects, increases their potency, and does not interfere with their cancer-killing action.

Adriamycin

As early as 1977, laboratory scientists noted that vitamin E does not interfere with Adriamycin's activity. (16, 304) When laboratory pigs were given vitamin E along with Adriamycin, they suffered less severe heart damage than those pigs that received Adriamycin alone. (167) In rabbits, heart muscle damage from Adriamycin was also lessened by giving them vitamin E (as well as vitamin A). (282) Many other laboratory studies revealed beneficial effects from adding vitamin E to Adriamycin treatment. (16, 101, 130, 141, 168, 190, 217, 284, 304, 305,314, 374, 406, 432, 433, 438, 456)

Overwhelmingly, such studies find that "vitamin E...enhances the growth inhibitory effects of Adriamycin...on a variety of cancer cells..." and "adds to tumor reduction and decreases metastasis."(473) In a study in Angora rabbits, vitamin E even showed an ability to prevent the hair loss associated with Adriamycin treatment. (356)

Vitamin E and Other Toxic Treatments

Another drug with which vitamin E has a positive interaction is 5-FU. Scientists at Vanderbilt University, describe the combination of vitamin E and 5-FU as "a novel therapy" for colon and rectal cancer." (65) Vitamin E protects against the ravages of the CMF drug combination (which contains 5-FU) by restoring membrane lipids (fats) to normal. (427) Rats receiving vitamin E supplements at the same time as 5-FU had levels of harmful oxidation that were "significantly lower than those which had received only the anticancer drug." (60)

Retinoic Acid

Vitamin E works well with 13-cis-retinoic acid (retinoic acid or 13cRA). Unlike the natural vitamin, retinoic acid is somewhat toxic. Used alone, it yields about 10 percent complete responses in oral pre-cancers.

In a clinical trial at M.D. Anderson Cancer Center, Houston, that figure leaped to 78 percent when vitamin E was added. (96)

Methotrexate

Vitamin E also increases the effectiveness and decreases the toxicity of another standard drug, methotrexate. (101) Methotrexate interferes with the ability of white blood cells to migrate in the human body. But four studies in Poland showed that vitamin E could prevent this ominous form of toxicity. (364, 365, 435,436) Conversely, there are no studies showing that vitamin E interferes with either the safety or effectiveness of methotrexate.

Cisplatin

Cisplatin is often toxic to the kidneys. Egyptian researchers found that vitamin E significantly reduced the toxicity of cisplatin in experimental animals. The levels of detoxification enzymes were also significantly increased by vitamin E.

It also partially reversed many of the kidney enzymes changes induced by cisplatin. The authors called this mixture a "promising compound for reducing cisplatin-toxic side effects" including kidney toxicity. (102) There are over a half dozen additional studies showing a beneficial effect when vitamin E is added to cisplatin, but none to my knowledge suggesting that it interferes. (18, 42, 60, 152, 181, 358, 399)

Vitamin E and Radiation

Does vitamin E interfere with the effects of radiation therapy? On the contrary, most studies have shown that vitamin E protects against radiation's side effects. In a series of experiments, dating back to the 1970s, scientists reported "a significantly enhanced effect of irradiation by tocopherol."(191, 192, 193) One study found that "injection of alpha-tocopherol immediately after irradiation significantly reduced radiation lethality."(261) Russian studies showed that vitamin E increased 30-day survival rates in irradiated animals. (385)

Scientists at the U.S. Armed Forces Institute of Radiobiology concluded that "survival was significantly increased in mice given vitamin E" along with radiation treatments. (420) These results have been confirmed five times. (104, 366, 388, 401, 422)

Mice receiving radiation to their salivary glands showed protective effects when they were given vitamin E at the same time. (125) Few things in science are unanimous and there happens to be one 1980 report that found no benefit from adding vitamin E to radiation. (379) But scientists at the University of Minnesota Medical School summarized the consensus opinion: vitamin E is a significant protector, whose effects include increased survival after whole-body irradiation, diminished digestive problems, and improved blood scores after irradiation. (113)

In the "Bible" of radiation therapy, *Principles and Practice of Radiation Oncology*, the authors state that "Vitamin E, vitamin C, and beta-carotene protect cellular membrane lipids from the action of radiation-produced [free] radicals by scavenging these radicals." (345) They then pass on to other matters—one sentence in a 2,341 page textbook!

In his experiments, Dr. Prasad used a standard experimental model of cancer cells to look at the effects of vitamin E alone or in combination with various standard treatments. (357)

Combinations of Vitamin E and Conventional Agents

Agent Used	Decrease in Cancer Growth
Vitamin E	47%
Bleomycin	46%
Bleomycin + vitamin E	71%
5-FU	37%
5-FU + vitamin E	85%
Adriamycin	58%
Adriamycin + vitamin E	88%
Cisplatin	57%
Cisplatin + vitamin E	82%

Thus, you can see that vitamin E alone had a pronounced effect on cancer cells, as potent as Bleomycin and 5-FU. Yet when vitamin and chemotherapy were given together there was an even better outcome.

There is no suggestion here or elsewhere that vitamin E does any harm to cancer patients.

Choice of Vitamin E Supplements

Dr. Prasad has also shown that there is one form of the vitamin that is particularly effective against cancer cells. This is **alpha tocopherol suc-**

cinate. At the same time, it is important to get a mixture of the four tocopherols. Whenever possible, get the natural kind. You can tell a synthetic product because it is designated with the prefix "dl-" or "RS-" on the label. Although synthetics are less expensive, they are generally less effective.

Toxicity?

Alpha-tocopherol is not very toxic and 2000 IU have been given for months without any sign of harm. However, less is known about the effects of the other tocopherols, especially when they are taken in isolation. In addition, vitamin E should not be taken with iron. In fact, iron supplements are not recommended except for people who definitely have iron deficiency anemia. Also, very high doses of vitamin E should not be taken alone without also taking vitamins A and C.

To summarize: People who consume a diet high in vitamin E have lower rates of cancer than those who don't. Conversely, a lower level of vitamin E intake has repeatedly been found to increase the risk of many kinds of cancer, including lung and prostate.

My recommendation is to take 200 IU of natural mixed tocopherols as well as 200 IU of alpha-tocopherol-succinate each day. People actively fighting cancer should take 400 to 600 IU of each item, but no more. These are the most effective forms of vitamin E for cancer prevention and treatment.

10. Tocotrienols

There is a lesser-known class of vitamin E compounds called tocotrienols. These are the forms of vitamin E found in palm oil, rice bran oil, and a few other foods. Tocotrienols are relatively new entries on the health food scene. But evidence is accumulating that they can reduce unwanted fats in the circulatory system, break down foreign proteins, decrease tissue swelling, and exert strong anti-oxidative properties. **There are also hints that tocotrienols exert an anticancer effect.**

- Western Ontario scientists have shown that tocotrienols inhibit the growth of breast cancer cells, even those that are not estrogen-receptor positive. This could be important for women whose cells are not responsive to fairly effective drugs like tamoxifen. There is a need for clinical trials of tocotrienols with Co Q10 and lipoic acid in breast cancer patients. (335)
- English doctors found that tocotrienols could inhibit the growth of many kinds of breast cancer cells. However, it was the gamma- and delta-fractions of tocotrienol that were the most effective. They state that "inhibition of the growth of breast cancer cells by tocotrienols could have important clinical implications...." (313)
- University of Wisconsin scientists have found that gamma-tocotrienols suppress breast cancer, melanoma, and leukemia cells. (287)

Chemically, tocotrienols are only slightly different from tocopherols, yet sometimes small differences lead to important biological effects.

Tocotrienols can move around cell membranes with even greater facility than the tocopherols and distribute themselves more evenly. They are also forty to sixty times more readily recycled than the tocopherols, so that a little tocotrienol goes a long way.

Tocotrienols are predominantly found in the bran portion of cereal grains, such as in oat, rice or wheat, as well as barley and palm oil. (418) Grape seed oil, known for its health-promoting properties, also contains significant amounts of tocotrienol. (330)

Perhaps the most abundant dietary source of tocotrienols for the consumer is rice bran oil. Rice bran oil is primarily used in upscale snack foods and in Japanese restaurants, because of its stability at high cooking temperatures and its pleasant flavor.

But how much you get from a single serving, and how much good it does you, is a matter of scientific debate.

Tocotrienols appear to be safe and natural agents, which we eat in small quantities all the time. But there are still a number of practical questions that need to be ironed out before tocotrienols could be recommended.

One problem is what scientists call "bioavailability." Does the amount you ingest actually get into your system? They seem to be less readily absorbed by the body than tocopherols.

They are also expensive. A bottle of 60 tocotrienol capsules (50 milligrams each) costs almost $40.00. Some doctors recommend 100 milligrams each morning for every person and another 100 milligrams each afternoon for those with a family (or personal) history of cancer. However, 200 milligrams will cost you around $2.75 per day.

To summarize: Tocotrienols are an overlooked part of the vitamin E family and a promising area of antioxidant research. I think it is too early to make a recommendation for the general public. However, it would be sensible for people actively fighting cancer to take 100 to 200 milligrams of mixed tocotrienols per day if they can afford it.

11. Glutathione and Glutamine

Glutathione is so important that it is found in every living creature on earth. In human beings, glutathione is mostly found in the liver, spleen, kidneys, and pancreas, where it performs essential biological functions. It protects against damage to proteins in the brain and for that reason is often classed among the "smart nutrients." It also protects the stomach lining against environmental toxins.

One cannot overestimate glutathione's importance. It is one of the master antioxidants, along with vitamins C and E, Co Q10, and lipoic acid. (335)

Glutathione has a crucial role in the body's immune defenses. A loss of glutathione leads to an increased susceptibility to free radicals. Glutathione protects us from the effects of a variety of toxic substances. (472)

Glutathione and chemotherapy

Does glutathione interfere with chemotherapy? Quite the opposite. In Italy, scientists experimented with a combination of 2,500 milligrams of glutathione and the toxic drugs cisplatin and cyclophosphamide.

In a clinical trial, 20 women with advanced ovarian cancer were treated with this mixture. There was a complete response rate of 55 percent, even in patients with very advanced disease. The average survival was 26.5 months and 5 patients were still alive and disease-free three years later. These results were considered very good, given the stage and type of the cancer.

In addition, the toxicity of this treatment was unexpectedly mild, without any kidney damage (a common side effect of cisplatin).

Italian scientists therefore concluded that glutathione has no "negative interference" with cisplatin or cyclophosphamide's activity, and might improve the therapeutic results. (252) There are other studies that support this same conclusion. (92, 93, 331)

Incidentally, cyclophosphamide is one of those "classical alkylating agents" that Dr. Dan Labriola and Dr. Robert Livingston claim is "vulnerable to interaction with antioxidants." On theoretical grounds they warn oncologists to "avoid concurrent administration" of such drugs and antioxidants. (222) Studies such as the above contradict these unsubstantiated warnings.

Supplements?

Glutathione *per se* is difficult to absorb and only people known to have very low levels are likely to benefit from supplements. If you do take supplements of glutathione, be sure to also take selenium and vitamin B2, as these augment its antioxidant activity.

Most people would do better to take supplements that indirectly increase or preserve glutathione levels. The least expensive of these is lipoic acid, 50 to 100 milligrams of which increases glutathione levels by 30 percent or more. Other popular glutathione-boosters are the amino acid cysteine or N-acetylcysteine (NAC).

> NAC is interesting in its own right. (455) In 1995, Italian researchers wrote that NAC "is currently considered one of the most promising cancer chemopreventive agents..."(6) There are many studies showing "an evident synergism" between Adriamycin and NAC. (86) Another study found that NAC protects against heart damage, bone marrow damage, hair loss, and metastasis. (85) A single study, in mice, suggested that NAC interfered with the antitumor activity of Adriamycin (395) and cisplatin (286) Otherwise, the data is very positive.

Cancer patients generally take 600 to 1,200 milligrams of NAC once per day with food. This is safe and effective, but expensive for daily use. An alternative is to take whey protein, which contains glutathione and cysteine, as well as cofactors lactoferrin and lactalbumin, both of which increase the conversion of cysteine to glutathione.

Glutamine and Conventional Therapy

Glutamine is an amino acid that is the most abundant protein building block in the body. Glutamine helps create glutathione in the body.

Tumors love glutamine and cannot live without it. Tumors act as "glutamine traps," depleting the patient's own glutamine stores. This results in the wasting syndrome known as cachexia. (417)

In the test tube, at least, tumors seem dependent on glutamine for their growth. And as late as 1990, scientists were still worrying that glutamine supplements would stimulate tumor growth or make tumors more resistant to treatment. (416) Needless to say, these preliminary findings and theoretical concerns deterred its use in the clinic setting. (208)

This point-of-view was challenged by Suzanne Klimberg, M.D., director of women's oncology at the University of Arkansas. She helped to pioneer a new attitude towards glutamine. Her results were contrary to the opinions of most doctors. (26) She found that glutamine actually decreased tumor growth through stimulation of the immune system. When given along with radiation and chemotherapy, glutamine did not promote tumors but protected patients and actually increased the effectiveness of conventional treatments. (208) This was quite a surprise.

After seven weeks, rats given glutamine supplements had smaller tumors than those not given this amino acid. In fact, tumor growth was decreased by 40 percent. And this was associated with a 2.5-fold increase in natural killer cell activity. (209)

Despite this scientific evidence, negative attitudes towards glutamine persist. I recently attended a medical conference at which a prominent cancer doctor warned his colleagues not to give their patients glutamine, because, according to his outdated views, it would promote tumor growth.

In a clinical trial at Brigham and Women's Hospital, Boston, doctors studied the effects of glutamine supplements on patients undergoing bone marrow transplantation. Half the patients were randomized to receive a high dose of glutamine.

The length of hospitalization was significantly shorter in glutamine-treated patients. In addition, "the incidence of positive microbial cultures and clinical infection was also significantly lower with glutamine supplementation." The clincher was that hospital charges were $21,095 less per patient in the glutamine-supplemented group compared with patients who received standard therapy! But the retail cost for megadoses of glutamine is less than $10.00 per day.

Most other clinical studies support the safety and efficacy of glutamine supplements. For patients in an intensive care unit in Great Britain, the savings from glutamine amounted to "only" $7,900 per patient.

Another double-blind randomized trial at the University of Kansas Medical Center also found benefit. The length of a hospital stay after bone marrow transplantation was significantly shorter (by 5.8 days) in patients receiving glutamine. Incidence of positive bacterial cultures and clinical infections also declined. (394a)

A clinical trial at the Royal London Hospital found similar, albeit somewhat smaller, benefits. " Glutamine was associated with a significant reduction in length of stay in surgical patients," they reported, with 45 days for conventionally treated patients and 30 days for the glutamine group. (355, 485) Another randomized trial at the Geisinger Medical Center in Danville, Pennsylvania, found that glutamine supplements "blunted" the negative effects of surgery. (185)

Glutamine and Mouth Sores

Most studies show that glutamine can also prevent damage to the mucous membranes of the mouth. In animal studies, glutamine reduced chemotherapy-associated mouth sores (stomatitis or mucositis).

In patients with colorectal cancer who were receiving 5-FU, there was a significant reduction in mouth sores as well as stomach and duodenal ulcers after the third course of chemotherapy, according to doctors at the University of Heidelberg. (89)

A study at the University of Minnesota was similarly positive. Twelve patients received toxic chemotherapy treatments. After oral supplements of glutamine, the duration of mouth sores decreased in 13 out of 14 patients. Their doctors concluded that **"oral supplementation with glutamine can significantly decrease the severity of chemotherapy-induced stomatitis, an important cause of morbidity in the treatment of patients with cancer."** (415)

In a 1998 study at the Mayo Clinic, Rochester, Minnesota, glutamine had a significant effect on mouth sores. The duration of mouth pain was 4.5 days less in patients who received glutamine supplements, compared to those who just received a placebo. Patients could also start eating regular foods four days earlier. Minnesota scientists described glutamine as **"a simple and useful measure to increase the comfort of many patients at high risk of developing mouth sores as a consequence of intensive cancer chemotherapy."** (12)

Oral glutamine also decreased the severity and duration of mouth sores in patients who received their own bone marrow as a transplant (autologous BMT). They needed morphine for pain for only five days, compared to 10.3 days for the group that received a placebo. (184, 327)

Glutamine and Methotrexate

Chemotherapy can cause severe depression of the immune system and increased susceptibility to infection. Rats who were recovering from chemotherapy were given a kind of glutamine in their diet. Other rats were kept on a glutamine-free diet. Harvard scientists found that dietary glutamine improved the immune status of rats recovering from the effects of the drug methotrexate. This immune-enhancing effect was more pronounced the longer the rats got the supplement. (380)

Scientists at the University of Arkansas implanted tumors in mice and then gave half of them a glutamine-enriched diet. The result was tumors had an increased susceptibility to chemotherapy, with a shrinkage of tumors in the glutamine group. Scientists concluded that glutamine enhances the effectiveness of antitumor drugs by making cancer cells more susceptible to chemotherapy. (380)

Human Study

Nine women with inflammatory breast cancer were given oral glutamine supplements at the same time as methotrexate. There was no toxicity from the glutamine and, astonishingly, **"no patient showed any sign of chemotherapy-related toxicity."** With one exception, all patients responded to the chemotherapy, and the average survival was 35 months. Arkansas scientists concluded that glutamine is safe and helps increase the effectiveness of methotrexate. (381)

Glutamine and Diarrhea

An Italian study shows that very large glutamine supplements (18 grams per day) counteracts diarrhea in patients receiving chemotherapy. (303)

Negatives?

There have also been a few studies that found no benefit in giving glutamine to relieve mouth sores, particularly after 5-FU therapy. (327) However, most studies have been quite positive.

To summarize: Glutathione and glutamine supplements are probably unnecessary for the average person trying to prevent cancer. However, most studies show that it is **extremely important** for cancer patients undergoing conventional treatments to receive glutamine supplements. If you are such a patient, you should bring the above clinical studies to the attention of your oncologist.

12. Lipoic Acid

Lipoic acid is an emerging player on the antioxidant scene. It was discovered in 1937 by scientists who noticed that bacteria needed some mysterious ingredient in potato extract to grow in a Petri dish. Lipoic acid thus began its career as the unromantic "potato growth factor." In 1951, biochemist Lester Reed isolated it and mapped its molecular structure. To do so, he processed ten tons of beef liver in order to produce just 30 milligrams of the purified substance.

What he found is called alpha-lipoic acid, lipoate, thioctic acid but most commonly just lipoic acid.

Lipoic acid has been used in Europe for many years to reverse the effects of mushroom poisoning. This is an indication of its power to protect the liver, which is important to cancer patients, who are trying to detoxify and protect their main organ of detoxification.

Lipoic acid is becoming much better known. (334) Lester Packer calls lipoic acid "the most powerful of all the antioxidants....a super-antioxidant that breaks many of the rules regarding antioxidant behavior. In fact, if I were to invent an ideal antioxidant, it would closely resemble lipoic acid, which does everything an antioxidant should do and more." (335)

Lipoic acid is certainly remarkable. It helps protect against three of the most common ailments of aging: stroke, heart disease and cataracts.

Prof. Bruce Ames of the University of California, Berkeley, has shown that feeding old rats lipoic acid, as well as another food supplement called carnitine, for a few weeks, restored their energy levels, decreased signs of aging, and boosted their ability to move around. (11)

Ames made headlines when he enabled old rats to act and appear like young rodent pups. While we should not expect any single nutrient to be a fountain of youth, we are certainly learning that **a judicious combination of antioxidants can delay the aging process,** with its attendant host of infirmities. And lipoic acid is central to that process.

In addition, lipoic acid is a team player, which boosts the activity of the entire antioxidant network. Thus, when you take lipoic acid you also increase your levels of vitamins E and C, coenzyme Q10, and glutathione.

Lipoic acid and glutathione

Lipoic acid is similar in function to glutathione and in fact boosts the body's levels of glutathione by 30 to 70 percent. (52)

"We had found a substance that could increase glutathione," Prof. Packer says of lipoic acid, "and ironically this 'miracle substance' was not discovered in the laboratory of a huge drug company at a cost of billions of dollars, but it was something that nature had created and had been available to us all along. The lesson to be learned from this experiece is that sometimes scientists can yield the best results when we stop trying to compete with nature or improve upon it, and instead try to understand it." (335)

Lipoic Acid and Cancer

Lipoic acid will probably turn out to have a role in the prevention and treatment of cancer, as part of the larger antioxidant network.

Lipoic acid can also regulate the expression of genes. We are often told that our genes are our fate. But even if you do have some defective genes, the good news is that you can regulate them through environmental factors, such as diet, supplements, and lifestyle. These external factors can influence whether we develop a particular disease, even if we are genetically predisposed to do so. (377) Lipoic acid can turn off the genes that accelerate cancer, without any signs of toxicity. And it does so at a reasonable cost.

For reasons that are not quite understood, people (390) or animals (196) with cancer absorb lipoic acid. Research has shown that rats given experimental cancers soaked up injected lipoic acid in their various organs. The life spans of these rats was extended by 25 percent. (197)

Lipoic Acid and Leukemia

By itself, lipoic acid did not have a significant effect on acute promyelocytic leukemia (APL) cells in the laboratory. Lipoic acid and the other antioxidants helped vitamin D3 to fight against this kind of cancer. (400) Talking of vitamin D3, I should caution the reader that there is a down side to this otherwise excellent vitamin. Large amounts can raise the body's calcium levels precipitously and this could damage the kidneys. (113) In general, one should stick to the RDA, which is 400 IU per day.

Lipoic Acid and Chemotherapy

Does lipoic acid interfere with chemotherapy? So far the combination has only been found to be beneficial. Rats with cancers were pretreated with lipoic acid. The animals were then given two standard drugs, cyclophosphamide (Cytoxan) and Vincristine. German scientists concluded that by lowering the toxic side effects of the drugs, they were able to increase the survival of the animals. There was no negative effect on the activity of this form of chemotherapy. (32)

With Cisplatin

One of the big problems with the drug cisplatin is that it can cause hearing loss or even deafness. Scientists at Southern Illinois University have shown that this is due to free radical damage of the inner ear. Rats were given either cisplatin, lipoic acid, both or neither. As suspected, cisplatin caused a significant reduction in natural antioxidants such as glutathione in the ear.

But when lipoic acid was added, the amount of glutathione remained about the same as in the control animals. Researchers concluded that cisplatin's ability to damage hearing could be corrected by the simple addition of lipoic acid. (382)

Side Effects

Does lipoic acid itself have side effects? A daily intake of 50 milligrams of lipoic acid produces no specific side effects. When the dose is increased, there may be some low toxicity, such as over-alertness or insomnia. Stomach upset is a possibility at higher amounts. In doses over 500 milligrams per day or more, a slight blood glucose lowering effect is observed. Some allergic skin reactions have also been reported in a few people at these high doses. However, there is no evidence that lipoic acid promotes mutations, birth defects, or cancer.

To summarize: Lipoic acid is a promising member of the antioxidant network. My recommendation is that every person take 50 milligrams per day of lipoic acid, and that past or present cancer patients take 100 milligrams in divided doses at meal times. It should be taken as part of an overall antioxidant program. There is no evidence that lipoic acid interferes with radiation or chemotherapy. Quite the opposite: it appears beneficial.

13. Coenzyme Q10

Coenzyme Q10 (Co Q10) is a vital link in the body's energy chain. First isolated in 1957, it is found in every human, indeed every living, cell. Our bodies cannot function without it. As levels of Co Q10 drop, so does one's general health. And when levels falls below 25 percent of normal, life itself becomes impossible. For that reason, some people call this compound "vitamin Q10," although that term has not been officially recognized.

Because Co Q10 is so ubiquitous in nature, scientists have also dubbed it ubiquinone. It has been the subject of over 5,000 scientific articles, more than 500 of them in the last two years alone.

While Co Q10 can be found in foods such as organ meats, wheat germ, rice bran, and eggs, to get therapeutic doses one needs to take it in the form of supplements, preferably along with selenium, glutathione, and L-carnitine.

Co Q10 is a fat-soluble molecule and flourishes along with the work-horse of fat-protecting molecules, vitamin E. It is very popular in Japan as a treatment for heart failure, angina, arrhythmias, and high blood pressure. It also has a role in cancer treatment.

Co Q10 was discovered by Prof. Fred L. Crane in 1957, but its medical properties were first intensively investigated by Karl Folkers, Ph.D., of the University of Texas. Dr. Folkers, who won the President's Medal of Science in 1990, wrote almost 200 scientific articles on Co Q10. Until his death in 1997 at the age of 91, he remained a persuasive advocate for wider recognition of Co Q10. I met him at a conference in Copenhagen just before his death. He came from the United States in a wheelchair to present his latest findings. Here was a man totally devoted to science and to human welfare! He told some wonderful anecdotes about friends who apparently were cured of cancer by relying primarily on Co Q10. But he was a good enough scientist to understand the need for more controlled trials, which he did more than anyone else to foster.

Co Q10 and Immunity

The first suggestion of a link between Co Q10 and the immune system came in the 1970s, when it was shown that old mice, which had weakened immune systems, could be partially restored to "immunological responsiveness" with this substance. (38)

Dr. Folkers found that Co Q10 could balance a crucial ratio of white blood cells that was often out of line in HIV-infected individuals, as well as some cancer patients. He cited the long-term symptom-free survival of several people with AIDS-related complex using supplements of Co Q10. (116, 120) Other scientists have suggested that Co Q10 might inhibit some of the harmful chemicals that are produced by tumors. (171)

Co Q10 as Cancer Treatment

What about Co Q10 as a cancer treatment? As early as 1968, Dr. Folkers and colleagues pointed out that there were low levels of Co Q10 in both rat and human cancer tissues. (404) Further studies revealed that breast cancer and multiple myeloma patients frequently had lower levels of Co Q10 than the general population. (117)

In France, "a correlation was shown between the intensity of the deficiency and the bad prognosis of the breast disease." (188)

Anecdotal evidence accumulated for 35 years of a beneficial effect of Co Q10 in cancer patients. Dr. Folkers often spoke about such patients, and suggested that Co Q10 "has allowed survival...for periods of 5 to 15 years." (116)

Co Q10 Clinical Trial

It was not until late 1993, however, that Dr. Folkers arranged the first clinical trial of Co Q10. At a clinic in Copenhagen, Denmark, doctors treated 32 patients with advanced, "high risk" breast cancer.

In addition to the appropriate surgery and conventional treatment, each patient was given 90 milligrams of Co Q10 per day. They also received other vitamins, minerals, antioxidants, and essential fatty acids, such as are found in fish oil.

On this regimen, 6 of the 32 patients showed partial tumor regressions. In advanced patients, this seems significant. Then in October, 1993, a strange thing happened: one of these six women, on her own, increased her dosage from 90 to 390 milligrams per day.

By the next month, her doctors wrote, **the tumor was no longer palpable and in the following month, a mammogram confirmed the disappearance of her tumor.**

After that, another woman in the group also increased her dose, this time to 300 milligrams. Her tumor also soon disappeared and a clinical examination revealed no evidence of the prior residual tumor, nor of distant metastases. The patient was in excellent clinical condition and there was no residual cancer. (253, 254)

In 1995, the same scientists reported on the treatment of three additional women with what they were now calling "vitamin Co Q10." Each received a daily oral dose of 390 milligrams. The results were also encouraging. Excitement was generated when multiple liver metastases of one 44-year-old woman disappeared, and no sign of metastases could be found elsewhere in her body.

Another woman showed no signs of a previously detected tumor in her chest after six months of Co Q10 treatment. The Danish doctors reported that her condition was "excellent." (68)

There are some deficiencies in this clinical trial: the small number of patients and also the fact that the women received other conventional and non-conventional treatments. Dr. Folkers was well aware of the study's limitations. However, he regarded it as a promising start to clinical studies, which could represent an important advance in the treatment of cancer, especially when combined with other approaches.

Co Q10 is a logical supplement for many people. Although it is relatively expensive, it is not so compared to other cancer treatments. Over a period of six weeks, one can work up to 390 milligrams. And there are no known side effects. Co Q10 should always be taken with some fat or oil for better absorption. There is some scientific research suggesting that a form of the coenzyme called Q-Gel has much better absorbency that the usual powdered Co Q10. (300)

There is also a test that can determine the levels of Co Q10 in the body from a single drop of blood. (116) However, currently, no American laboratory offers this test. Thus, supplementation with fairly high amounts is the most prudent course.

Vitamin B6

There is a less expensive way to increase Co Q10 blood levels. In three tests, Co Q10 increased when patients also took a supplement of vitamin B6, or pyridoxine, together with the coenzyme. Folkers and his colleagues concluded that such increases were "clinically important." (452)

Selenium

In addition, it has been shown that a selenium deficiency lowers the level of Co Q10 by about 50 percent in the liver and 15 percent in the hearts of experimental animals. Since a daily intake of 200 micrograms of selenium is optimal for most people, it would be wise to make sure you get this much to maintain Co Q10 levels. One ounce per day of fresh Brazil nuts also supplies approximately this much selenium.

Co Q10 and Adriamycin

Co Q10 is chemically similar to Adriamycin. But while Co Q10 naturally protects heart cells from damage, Adriamycin damages the heart by competing with Co Q10. As early as 1976, it was shown that Co Q10 could protect against the heart-damaging effects of Adriamycin. Co Q10 supplements were called "indispensable" to the healthy functioning of the heart muscle in both rabbits and humans. (77)

It was thus logical to try Co Q10 in patients receiving Adriamycin. By giving Co Q10 supplements of 100 milligrams, doctors were able to prevent, or even reverse, the usual heart toxicity of Adriamycin. (34)

This heart protection could have a profound effect on survival. In 1977, scientists demonstrated a dramatic effect in mice with cancer. When they gave them Adriamycin alone, between 36 to 42 percent survived. But when they added Co Q10 to Adriamycin, the survival rate soared to between 80 and 86 percent. (83)

This work was extended to humans. It was shown that Co Q10 did not reduce the anti-tumor activity of Adriamycin. (451) Ten children with leukemia (ALL) and non-Hodgkin's lymphoma had their hearts protected from Adriamycin by Co Q10. (80) Such results have been confirmed almost a dozen times; **in no case has there been a suggestion that Co Q10 interferes with the effectiveness of Adriamycin.** (33, 66, 67, 76, 118, 119, 177, 205, 321, 324, 391) A combination of carnitine and Co Q10 exerted an even greater protective effect against Adriamycin than either alone. (84)

Negative? One study showed that Co Q10 protected lung cancer cells from radiation, but only at extremely high levels of the coenzyme. (256a)

To summarize: Co Q10 is an essential ingredient of life and has multiple health-giving effects. It is especially important for cancer patients. Extensive laboratory and clinical tests have shown that it does not undermine the anti-cancer effects of chemotherapy. Rather, it spares the normal tissues from the drugs' toxicity and therefore improve overall results.

Every person on an antioxidant program should take a supplement of Co Q10. The amount needed varies, but ranges from 30 to 390 milligrams, for those who are aggressively fighting the disease.

14. Pycnogenol® and Grape Seed Extract

Pycnogenol® is the proprietary name of a product derived from the bark of the French maritime pine tree (*Pinus maritima*). This bark contains about forty different antioxidant chemicals, called bioflavonoids. The bioflavonoids were discovered by my mentor Albert Szent-Györgyi, M.D., Ph.D., soon after he isolated ascorbic acid.

In the 1930s, Szent-Györgyi recognized that bioflavonoids had a special relationship to vitamin C, the first suggestion that antioxidants work better when they are taken in combination. This intuitive insight was only confirmed 60 years later. (336)

A Warning on Tangeretin

While bioflavonoids are generally nontoxic, there is a potential danger in isolating one such substance and taking it in this isolated form. For instance, it has been found in animals that a bioflavonoid in citrus fruit, called tangeretin, inhibits the activity of the drug tamoxifen. (46)

There is no data yet to suggest that the same thing happens in people. However, I consider this a warning flag and feel that high amounts of tangeretin should be avoided by patients who are also taking tamoxifen.

Tangeretin may exert this negative effect by inhibiting natural killer cell activity. Drinking orange juice and eating citrus fruits is fine, and small amounts (around 25 to 50 milligrams) of citrus bioflavonoids in a multivitamin pill are unlikely to do any harm. But avoid foods with added citrus oils and especially avoid taking dietary supplements of citrus bioflavonoids themselves, especially if you are taking tamoxifen.

The dose that is possibly harmful to humans is 280 milligrams per day. Until there is more definitive data in humans, I recommend that people taking tamoxifen avoid taking high-dose supplements of citrus bioflavonoids.

Many of the ingredients in Pycnogenol have now been isolated and studied, but it has greater effects as a mixture than its purified components do individually, since the components work together synergistically. (64)

This synergism was seen in a 1999 study from Tokyo. Ophthalmologists looking for ways to prevent damage to the retina of the eye concluded that Pycnogenol was the most powerful of all the antioxidants they studied. It protected the retina 61 percent of the time. And when it was combined with vitamin E and coenzyme Q10 this excellent result was even further enhanced. (462)

Pycnogenol also refreshes vitamin C in the body and protects glutathione and vitamin E from free radical damage. It boosts the level of vitamin E by 15 percent. (63) Pycnogenol also increase natural killer cell cytotoxicity. (318) For that reason alone Pycnogenol could play an important role in immune and circulatory disorders, as well as diseases of the nervous system. (318)

Pycnogenol is said to be 20 times as potent an antioxidant as vitamin C and 50 times more potent than vitamin E. Lester Packer has said, **"of all the natural compounds tested in my laboratory for antioxidant activity, Pycnogenol is the strongest."** It can quench three kinds of free radicals, including the one that is most dangerous since it can directly attack DNA. The only substance that exceeds it at scavenging free radicals is green tea extract. (376) Pycnogenol is easily assimilated and put to use.

Crossing the Blood-Brain Barrier

The powerful antioxidants in Pycnogenol can pass through the blood-brain barrier, and are therefore able to protect the brain from free radical damage. For this reason, it is widely used to boost memory and fight senility. Scientists at Loma Linda Medical School in California have proposed Pycnogenol for the prevention of disorders associated with aging. (251) They fed Pycnogenol to old, semi-senile mice. After two months there was a significant improvement in the ability of their old bones to create new white blood cells. They concluded that Pycnogenol could be useful to either retard aging or restore the signs of youth. (176)

Smokers Take Note

Pycnogenol was able to prevent the formation of a carcinogen called NNK, derived from tobacco smoke. University of Michigan researchers concluded that orally ingested Pycnogenol may afford protection against lung tumors caused by NNK. (257)

Grape Seed Extract

A compound very similar in composition to Pycnogenol is grape seed extract. It also contains a high proportion of anthocyanins. Although Pycnogenol was the first anthocyanin supplement to appear in the United States, grape seed extract (depending on the brand) is usually more potent, containing between 92 to 95 percent bioflavonoids, compared to 85 percent for Pycnogenol.

Cost

Grape seed extract is considerably less expensive than Pycnogenol. It is available for about 20¢ per tablet. Look for brands that are manufactured using water and ethanol, without the use of synthetic solvents. **For a less expensive way of adding grape seed extract to your diet, try eating the seeds of organic red grapes.** There are anticancer substances in grape skins, the grapes themselves, but especially the seeds. Don't throw away the most valuable parts. And avoid seedless varieties when you shop.

To summarize: Pycnogenol and grape seed extract are certainly powerful mixtures of antioxidants. Although little research has been done on their relationship to cancer, they can be a useful part of an aggressive antioxidant program.

15. Selenium

Selenium (Se) is a metal that is chemically similar to sulfur. It was first discovered in 1817 and because of its silvery color was named for Selene, the ancient goddess of the moon.

Selenium is an essential component of two important antioxidant enzymes and is also the helpmate of vitamin E. Common food sources include garlic, onions, wheat germ, broccoli, and egg yolks, although the amount of selenium in food varies greatly depending on its concentration in the soil in which the food was grown. For many reasons, including the prevention of cancer, it is very important to maintain adequate levels of selenium.

Initially, selenium's importance in human health was underrated. In fact, its main use in conventional medicine was as a treatment for dandruff! One of the pioneers of selenium research was Emanuel Revici, M.D., an unconventional cancer doctor in New York who championed combinations of selenium and organic compounds for decades. It slowly worked its way from alternative to conventional medicine, mainly due to the work of Dr. Gerhard Schrauzer and his colleagues at the University of California, San Diego.

They performed many important studies on the protective effects of selenium. In one, they compared feeding typical American, Bulgarian, and Japanese diets to mice with breast cancer. The rate of breast cancer in mice receiving the antioxidant-rich Bulgarian diet was 27 percent of the mice fed a typical American diet. The "Japanese mice" scored somewhere in the middle, because most of their selenium came from a less easily assimilated source. But the best results came when the "Japanese mice" were given selenium supplements. Then, their rate of breast cancer fell to just 10 percent that of the "American mice." (395)

Other early clues to selenium's power came from studies of soil composition. In the 1960s, Dr. Raymond J. Shamberger found that **people who lived in states that have the lowest amounts of selenium in their soil are three times more likely to die of heart disease than inhabitants of states with selenium-rich soil.**

The selenium-poor states included Connecticut, Illinois, Ohio, Oregon, Massachusetts, Rhode Island, New York, Pennsylvania, Indiana and Delaware, as well as the District of Columbia. Incidentally, the city of Colorado Springs, Colorado has the highest selenium content in its soil of any city in the United States and one of the lowest death rates from heart disease. This has to be more than coincidental.

These surprising findings were then confirmed in other places in the world whose soils were selenium poor, such as Finland. Scientists concluded that "selenium supplementation may in subjects with low selenium reduce the risk of coronary heart disease." (403)

More recently, Chinese scientists showed that selenium is also able to cure Keshan's disease, which is initially triggered by a virus that attacks the heart. Vitamin E is similarly effective. These nutrients suppress the genes that are essential for the virus to spread. So here is another example of our environment, in this case selenium and vitamin E supplements, proving themselves able to control "bad genes."

Dr. Raymond Shamberger was also among the first to discover the link between low selenium content in the soil and increasing numbers of deaths from cancer. In 1976, **he pointed out that the cities and states with high selenium content in the soil also had significantly lower rates of cancer, especially of the digestive and urinary systems.** (471)

The Garlic Connection

It has long been noted that people who ate garlic, onion, broccoli, and whole grains had a reduced risk of cancer. It turns out that all of these foods are rich in selenium. In fact, selenium is one of the reasons that these particular foods are so healthful for us.

The Willett Study

Walter C. Willett of Harvard School of Public Health, Boston, has done much of the work that associates low selenium levels with higher cancer rates. In 1973, he and his colleagues took blood samples from 4,480 seemingly healthy American men. Their health was then monitored for the next five years and during this time, 111 of the men developed cancer. Their blood was then compared to that of men who did not develop cancer. (471)

The selenium levels in the blood of the cancer patients was significantly lower than in the non-cancer individuals. In fact, the risk of cancer in those having the least amount of selenium in their blood was double that of men with the highest levels. Again, this association was strongest for cancers of the digestive tract and the prostate. (78)

In the following year, scientists at Cornell University, Ithaca, New York, showed that people with the lowest levels of serum selenium had not just double, but a 5.8 times greater odds of getting skin cancer than those with the highest levels. This study was to have an astonishing and unexpected outcome. At the National Cancer Institute (NCI), this work stirred great interest. NCI therefore sponsored a study at seven dermatology clinics to see if selenium supplements could indeed prevent skin cancer.

Over 1,300 patients with a history of the most common kinds of skin cancer were given either a supplement of selenium (200 micrograms per day of selenium-enriched yeast) or a placebo pill.

Participants were then followed for eight years. At the end of this trial, it was found that selenium had no effect on the rate of skin cancer. However, disappointed scientists then began to study the rates for other kinds of cancer, and were amazed by what they found.

The group taking selenium had half the death rate from the far more serious internal cancers, such as those of the lung, colon, rectum, and prostate than the placebo group. (71) There was no toxicity from selenium at this level.

Supplements of selenium costs pennies a day, are harmless, and in this study prevented half the deaths from the most common cancers.

The selenium treatment was associated with an even more significant 63 percent reduction in prostate cancer incidence. The effect was even greater when scientists excluded people who already had high prostate-specific antigen (PSA) scores going into the trial. High PSAs are often indicative of pre-existing prostate problems, including sometimes cancer. When the high PSA volunteers were excluded, there were four times as many cases of prostate cancer in the placebo group as in the treatment group. (70, 479)

In another study, carried out by the Peking Union Medical College in Beijing, China, selenium-enriched table salt was given to people in an area (Qidong county) where there is both a low level of selenium in the soil and high rates of hepatitis B infection and primary liver cancer. This study involved over 130,000 people in the general population.

Half of these people were given selenium supplements. After 8 years, there was a reduction in primary liver cancer incidence by over 35 percent. Once the selenium-enriched table salt was withdrawn, the incidence of liver cancer began to rise again. However, the inhibition of hepatitis B was sustained during this withdrawal period.

People who have positive blood markers for hepatitis B are at a high risk of liver cancer. In each group, there were 113 people with such markers. In the placebo group, seven of these progressed to liver cancer, whereas none of those in the selenium supplement group did so. This protective effect disappeared when the selenium was withdrawn. Chinese scientists concluded that "a continuous intake of selenium is essential to sustain the chemopreventive effect." (71)

You might think that these astonishing findings would lead our medical leaders to embrace the idea of selenium supplementation. After all, no study has suggested that 200 micrograms per day of selenium is harmful. Yet these results, published in the *Journal of the American Medical Association* on Christmas Day, 1996, were accompanied by an editorial that sounded the tired old note that people should not begin taking selenium supplements. "These effects of selenium require confirmation...before new public health recommendations regarding selenium supplementation can be made," they wrote. (413)

Follow-up research will take a decade or more, if it ever happens, and if history is any guide, will be followed by yet more calls for further research. There is no end to research. In the meantime, however, millions more people will die of cancers that might have been prevented with a pill that costs pennies. Wouldn't it make more sense to say that our provisional recommendation is that every adult take 200 micrograms per day? I think Dr. Robert Atkins' acerbic comment is fully justified: "Needless to say, drug studies aren't greeted with such hesitation so routinely."

Laboratory studies

Laboratory studies have shown that selenium can inhibit the growth of breast, cervical, colon, and skin cancer. (179, 175, 372, 51).

Selenium and Chemotherapy

Does selenium interfere with radiation and chemotherapy? Once again, the evidence says, No.

Human ovarian tumor cells were exposed to a low concentration of the chemotherapy drug melphalan (L-PAM). They quickly developed resistance and could no longer be killed by the drug. But when low levels of selenium were included in the test tube, this "completely prevented the development of resistance." Rutgers University scientists concluded that this compound "may prove to be useful in preventing the development of drug resistance" in people as well. (55, 56)

In an animal study, human ovarian tumor cells that had been

pretreated with melphalan were injected into mice: the resulting tumors were rendered resistant to the drug. The mice were then treated with selenium. This treatment resulted in a decrease in the rate of growth of tumors. (430)

In a human study in Finland, 41 women with cancer were given supplements of selenium and/or vitamin E. Selenium decreased the toxicity of chemotherapy. Scientist concluded that **"selenium supplementation might thus be beneficial during cytotoxic [cell-killing] chemotherapy in ovarian cancer patients with low selenium levels."** (408, 429)

In Poland, scientists studied the effects of antioxidants in women undergoing chemotherapy for ovarian cancer. Each woman was given a daily dose of 200 micrograms of selenium (as well as other antioxidants.) Polish scientists concluded that "the administration of selenium in patients with ovarian cancer undergoing multi-drug chemotherapy is recommended." (482)

Selenium and Brain Cancer

It is known that selenium accumulates in tumor tissue more than in normal brain tissue. (338) It seems more than coincidental that many of Dr. Revici's most successful cases were patients with brain cancer.

At a hospital in Germany, doctors carried out a clinical trial on the effect of selenium in 32 brain cancer patients. These men and women were no longer responding to conventional treatment. All had increased pressure inside their heads, a typical sign of brain cancer.

Selenium levels were found to be abnormally low in 70 percent of these patients. All patients were given high-dose injections of selenium for up to eight weeks, in addition to some other non-conventional treatments.

Seventy-six percent of the patients showed "definite improvement" and the rest of them had "slight improvement" in such symptoms as nausea, vomiting, headache, vertigo, unsteady gait, speech disorders, and seizures. The German doctors concluded that selenium "can be employed with... other supportive measures in the management of brain tumor patients." (186)

Selenium and Chemoradiation

A study done in Tübingen, Germany showed that selenium given by mouth did not undo the effects of chemotherapy plus radiation. Patients with advanced rectal cancer were treated with a combination of selenium, the drug 5-FU, and radiation. Scientists reported a protective effect of selenium on quality of life.

"Our data show that oral selenium intake in rectal cancer patients is easily tolerated with no side effects," they wrote, while emphasizing the need for larger studies. (155)

Chinese Studies

There is a Chinese mixture of selenium and wheat germ that increases the presence of a substance called MT (metallothionein) in the liver and kidneys. (See the next chapter on zinc for a fuller explanation of MT.) Some doctors had feared that by increasing MT they might also increase the resistance of cancer cells to the drug cisplatin. However, in this experiment, the mixture "did not affect the anticancer activity" of cisplatin. The MT levels were "not increased in cancer" and also "did not cause drug-resistance of cancer cells." (475)

Dose

The Recommended Daily Allowance (RDA) is 50 to 100 micrograms (*not milligrams!*) but few people get even that much. Selenium is so important that I believe that practically every adult should take a 200 microgram selenium supplement every day. This is readily available in health food stores at a minimal price. Organic selenium derived from yeast may be better absorbed than the mineral form, sodium selenite. Very high doses of either can be toxic, however, and should only be taken under a doctor's prescription.

To summarize: Selenium has a strong ability to prevent cancers, especially of the internal organs. There is no evidence that selenium interferes with chemotherapy, radiation or a combination of both. On the contrary, there is evidence that it decreases the side effects of such treatments.

16. Zinc

Zinc is a mineral that is required in very small amounts by the human body. Zinc plays a crucial role in the formation of powerful antioxidants, especially vitamin A. (425, 443) An adequate intake of zinc is necessary to prevent a variety of diseases, including, according to the latest research, cancer.

There are now almost 3,000 articles documenting the relationship of zinc to cancer. Some show that a lack of zinc in the diet is associated with higher rates of cancer. In a now famous experiment, zinc supplements (given together with vitamin A) had a profound effect on the death rate from cancers of the esophagus and stomach, as well as cancers in general.

Some laboratory experiments have suggested that zinc has an anti-cancer role. For example, when scientists gave the carcinogenic mineral cadmium to rats, they developed cancer in their testes. But a lack of zinc in the diet increased the rate at which such cancer developed. NCI scientists concluded that "dietary zinc deficiency appears to cause a generalized increase in the chronic toxic effects of cadmium." (463)

Prostate cancer patients also have lower blood levels of zinc than patients with a non-malignant prostate condition. (229)

The Linxian Experiment

The most dramatic demonstration of zinc's preventive power came in the mid-1990s from a large study carried out in Linxian, China. Linxian province has the dubious distinction of being the "world capital" of cancer of the esophagus and upper stomach. There are numerous theories about what causes these skyrocketing rates. One theory is that the soil in this province lacks zinc and selenium, and that consequently the people do not get enough of these crucial minerals in their food.

For years, Chinese cancer scientists worked with U.S. researchers to find a solution to this terrible scourge. Together, they devised a large test to see if giving residents supplements could lower the death rates from these two kinds of cancer. In China, because of the size of the population and the aggressive public health policies of the government, it is possible to do very large studies: this particular one had 30,000 participants.

Between 1982 and 1991, combinations of various food supplements were given to volunteers. The dosages were from two to three times the

Recommended Daily Allowances. What they discovered was nothing less than astounding. **Stomach cancer among those who received the zinc and vitamin A combination was decreased by an astonishing 62 percent compared to those who did not receive these supplements.**

In addition, **a combination of beta-carotene, vitamin E, and selenium caused a 42 percent reduction in esophageal cancer.** People receiving supplements had lower overall cancer death rates as well. (233) This included a reduction in overall deaths by 9 percent; cancer deaths by 13 percent; stomach cancer deaths by 20 percent; and deaths from all other cancers by 19 percent.

I can only guess at what these scientists said privately about their ability to reduce esophageal cancer by 42 percent with a simple vitamin-mineral pill. Publicly they merely called this study "a hopeful sign" which "should encourage additional studies...in larger numbers of subjects." (216)

But many people need to make decisions about supplementation now.
They cannot wait for additional studies,
which invariably lead to calls for even further studies.

Moderate doses of zinc, beta-carotene, selenium and vitamin E are safe and inexpensive. I believe these results are valid and are an accurate reflection of what antioxidants can do. The finding that two terrible cancers could be prevented by a few pennies worth of supplements received little attention in the mainstream media.

Mouth Cancer

In 1995, scientists in India published a study on the use of a four-supplement pill—zinc, vitamin A, the B vitamin riboflavin, and selenium. Smoking is known to cause breaks in the genetic material (DNA). The scientists wanted to understand the effects of this supplement pill on the broken DNA of heavy smokers. Out of nearly 300 volunteers, half were given the supplement pill and half a placebo.

The results were striking. **At the end of one year, the frequency of DNA breaks decreased by 72 to 95 percent in the supplement group.** No such effects were seen in the placebo group.

There were complete remissions in 57 percent of the people who received supplements, while only 8 percent of those receiving the placebo showed a similar response. (361)

The Indian scientists' mild conclusion was that DNA damage "appears to be modifiable by the administration of micronutrient supplements." (100)

Zinc, MT and Chemotherapy

Scientific opinion is divided on the advisability of taking zinc supplements while undergoing chemotherapy, however. The question hinges on the activity of a class of compounds called MT (metallothioneins). These play an important role in regulating metals in the body. As background: some metals, like zinc, are necessary in small amounts but in large amounts they can be toxic. For example, some people have gotten sick to their stomachs by consuming acidic foods or drink that have been stored in a galvanized (zinc-lined) container.

Because too much metal is bad for us, the body has evolved ingenious ways of regulating its presence with substances called metallothioneins. A metallothionein is a small protein, rich in sulfur-containing amino acids, that is made in the liver and kidneys in response to the presence of metals such as zinc, mercury, cadmium, and copper, and that binds them tightly, rendering them harmless.

Why is this of concern in cancer chemotherapy? Because there is one type of anticancer drug that has a metal, platinum, at its core. Both cis-platinum and carbo-platinum are routinely used in chemotherapy today. While other forms of chemotherapy are probably unaffected, it is possible that MT decreases the toxicity of platinum-containing drugs. This concern is largely hypothetical.

It does not appear to be valid in the case of brain cancer. Scientists at the University of California, San Francisco put rodents with brain cancer on a high-zinc diet. They then increased the dose of carboplatin by 50 percent without increased damage to the bone marrow. Nor was there any reduction in the effectiveness of carboplatin against this experimental brain tumor. (100) It would probably take a very high level of zinc to interfere with this type of chemotherapy. (328)

A clinical trial in China studied the effects of a zinc-and-licorice mixture on chemotherapy. Mice were given this combination as well as cisplatin. The mixture significantly reduced kidney, blood, and testicular toxicity. At the same time, the mixture did not undermine chemotherapy either in the animals or in the test tube. (475a)

Another Chinese trial studied immune reactions in cancer patients receiving zinc and selenium supplements. Immune skin reaction were strengthened, white blood cells became healthier, and interferon levels were increased by both zinc and a combination of zinc and selenium.

Chinese scientists concluded that zinc was instrumental in restoring failing immune systems in cancer patients. (273)

Another clinical trial incorporating zinc into cancer treatment showed promising results. Prior to surgery, Mexican doctors gave 20 patients with squamous cell cancers of the head and neck a combination of zinc, the standard anticancer drug cyclophosphamide, and indomethacin, as well as an immune-stimulating mixture.

Eighteen out of twenty patients showed a reduction of their tumors by 44 percent, as well as a desirable infiltration of tumor by white blood cells. This "indicates immunization to the tumor," they wrote. (480) It is impossible to know the relative importance of the various agents employed. However, there was no suggestion that zinc undermined the therapeutic goal: quite the opposite, these results appeared due to the synergism of cytotoxic with immune-boosting agents, such as zinc.

Overall, the fear that zinc or MT will undo the effects of platinum-containing drugs seems largely hypothetical. To err on the side of caution, you could suspend zinc supplements while taking cisplatin or carboplatin.

Zinc and Radiation Therapy

Zinc can be used to protect against damage from radiation therapy. In animal experiments, when zinc was added to the synthetic antioxidant Amifostine, the effect was greater than with Amifostine alone. (115)

To summarize: Zinc is an essential part of the antioxidant program. Every person trying to prevent cancer should be sure to get a daily supply. Although zinc is found in a number of foods, many people do not get the small Recommended Daily Allowance (RDA). This fact alone argues strongly for taking supplements that contain zinc, along with other nutrients. Zinc supplements are safe and are a good "insurance policy" for almost everybody.

For basic prevention most people will do well with 15 to 25 milligrams. Higher doses should only be taken under the guidance of a health professional. Zinc tends to compete for uptake with other minerals, such as copper, manganese and iron. Taking more than 200 milligrams per day could contribute to deficiencies of these other minerals.

Zinc should be taken at a different time than other supplements and not with meals, as some foods (soy, cow's milk, whole wheat bread, etc.) may interfere with its absorption.

17. *Melatonin*

What is the most powerful antioxidant? In a comparative study, vitamin C, vitamin E, and glutathione all yielded the laurels to melatonin. (292) Melatonin is a product of the pineal gland in the brain. It is a hormone, but is sold over the counter in the U.S. In some countries, such as Canada, it is available by prescription only.

Its main medical use is to counteract insomnia and jet lag. However, some scientists have begun to use it in cancer therapy, as well.

The usual dose for inducing sleep is between 0.5 and 3 milligrams per night. But in the clinical studies about to be described, the therapeutic dose was usually 20 milligrams taken by mouth in the evening.

The great name in this field is Dr. Paolo Lissoni. Together with colleagues at San Gerardo Hospital, Milan, Italy, he has written over 100 scientific articles and performed about a dozen rigorous randomized clinical trials using this substance. I will briefly summarize them.

Lung Cancer

Dr. Lissoni and his colleagues tested melatonin in 63 people with metastatic non-small cell lung cancer whose tumors had grown while receiving cisplatin. Thirty-one of these patients were given melatonin and the rest received no further cancer treatment. More people were alive at one year who were treated with melatonin than the others. There were no major side effects to the melatonin, and in fact the patients' quality of life improved while on the hormone. (240, 368)

In his later studies, Dr. Lissoni combined melatonin with low doses of the immune stimulants interleukin-2 (IL-2) and interferon-alpha. These are both FDA-approved drugs that have to be prescribed by a physician.

Melatonin and IL-2

In this study, 20 patients with lung cancer were given 10 milligrams per day of melatonin as well as injected doses of IL-2. A partial response was achieved in four out of twenty patients. Ten others had their disease stabilized, while six patients had no benefit from the treatment. (237)

Melatonin and Chemotherapy

In another study, 60 patients with locally advanced or metastatic non-small cell lung cancer were randomized to receive either immunotherapy (with IL-2 and melatonin) or chemotherapy, consisting of cisplatin and etoposide. No complete response was obtained in either group. Roughly equivalent results were achieved in the two groups, with partial responses in 7 out of 29 patients treated with chemotherapy and in 6 out of 31 patients receiving chemotherapy. But both progression-free periods and overall one-year survivals were higher in the immunotherapy group than in those treated with chemotherapy. Predictably, toxicity was substantially lower in patients receiving immunotherapy than in those given chemotherapy. (249)

More on Lung Cancer

The Milan scientists also carried out another randomized clinical trial of chemotherapy alone vs. chemotherapy plus melatonin in advanced non-small cell lung cancer patients who had a poor clinical status.

This study included 70 advanced lung cancer patients who received cisplatin and etoposide or this chemotherapy plus melatonin. One patient's tumor completely disappeared when treated with chemotherapy plus melatonin. That was not the case with any of the patients receiving chemotherapy alone.

Ten patients (out of 34) who received melatonin had partial shrinkages of their tumors. Only 6 out 36 chemotherapy patients responded in this way. Thus, the tumor response rate was higher in patients receiving melatonin (11 out of 34) than in those who did not receive it (6 out of 35).

The percentage of patients who survived at least one year was twice as great in patients treated with melatonin plus chemotherapy than in those who received chemotherapy alone.

Chemotherapy was well tolerated in patients receiving melatonin, and the frequency of blood marrow suppression, nerve damage, and the wasting syndrome (cachexia) was significantly lower in the melatonin group. **This study showed that melatonin could improve the effectiveness of standard chemotherapy both in terms of survival and reduced drug toxicity.** (247)

Breast Cancer with Epirubicin

Melatonin inhibits the proliferation of human breast cancer cells in culture. It also increases antioxidant levels in breast cancer cells and reduces estrogen receptors on breast cancer cells. Since estrogen effectively feeds the growth of hormone-responsive breast tumors, "reducing the receptors might slow tumor growth," according to *Science News* (7/3/93).

In a human clinical trial with melatonin and the drug epirubicin, there were superior results compared to the use of either agent alone. In women with advanced breast cancer, who got both agents, tumor shrinkages were seen in 5 out of 12 (or 41 percent) of the patients. Other studies have repeatedly shown a decrease in toxicity with, at the very least, no loss of effectiveness. (250, 291, 298, 368)

Breast Cancer with Tamoxifen

Melatonin was evaluated as a treatment for women with metastatic breast cancer whose tumors had grown while they were taking the hormonal drug tamoxifen. A partial response was achieved in 4 out of 14 (28.5 percent) patients, with an average length of eight months. The treatment was well tolerated in all cases, and there was no enhancement of tamoxifen's toxicity. On the contrary, most patients experienced a relief of anxiety. Serum levels of insulin-like growth factor 1 (IGF-1), a tumor-promoting hormone, significantly decreased on this combined therapy, and the decline was significantly higher in those who responded to the treatment. (25, 248)

Colorectal

There was a randomized clinical trial of melatonin and low-dose IL-2 in 50 metastatic colorectal cancer patients, who were no longer responding to the standard drug 5-FU. Patients received either supportive care alone or the combined melatonin-IL-2 treatment. 3 out of 25 patients treated with melatonin and IL-2 had partial tumor shrinkages. Three times as many of these patients were alive at one year compared with those who were treated with supportive care alone. (244)

Primary Brain

This randomized clinical trial included 30 patients with a kind of brain cancer, glioblastoma, who received radiation therapy alone, or radiation plus melatonin. The percent of patients surviving one year was significantly higher in patients treated with radiation plus melatonin than in those receiving radiation alone (6 out of 14 vs. 1 out of 16). Moreover, radiation or steroid-related toxicity was less frequent in patients also receiving melatonin. (246)

Stomach

In a small study of 14 patients with stomach cancer, a partial regression was achieved in 3 out of 14 (21 percent). There was a complete disappearance of the tumor in one of these patients. The average length of these responses was more than 13 months. (235)

All Types Combined

In the largest randomized clinical trial, Dr. Lissoni gave 80 consecutive patients with advanced cancer either IL-2 alone or IL-2-plus-melatonin. (Two tumor types, melanoma and renal cancer, were excluded for technical reasons.) A complete response was obtained in 3 out of 41 patients treated with IL-2 plus melatonin and in none of the patients receiving IL-2 alone. A partial response was achieved in 8 out of 41 patients treated with IL-2 plus melatonin but in only 1 out of 39 patients treated with IL-2 alone. The number of patients whose tumors shrank was 27 percent in those getting both treatments. Such patients also had a higher one-year survival rate of 46 percent compared to 15 percent in those receiving only IL-2. (238, 239, 241)

Brain Metastases

Another clinical trial included 50 patients who were randomly assigned to receive either supportive care alone or supportive care plus melatonin. Survival without any sign of tumor growth at one year, as well as the average survival time, were both significantly higher in patients treated with melatonin than in those who received supportive care alone. Complications and side effects were significantly more frequent in patients treated with supportive care alone than in those also treated with melatonin. (239)

Melanoma

Thirty relapsed melanoma patients were randomized to receive either no treatment or adjuvant therapy with melatonin every day until there were signs of the disease progressing. At 31 months, the percent of patients with disease-free survival was significantly higher in the melatonin-treated individuals than in the controls. They also survived longer. No melatonin-related toxicity was observed. (298)

Cachexia

Melatonin has also been tested as a way of preventing the wasting syndrome of advanced cancer called cachexia. There were 86 evaluable patients. Although there was no difference in food intake, the percentage of serious weight loss was significantly less in patients treated with melatonin plus supportive care than in those who received supportive care alone. (245)

Melatonin with Chemotherapy

Melatonin is another antioxidant that protects against the side effects of chemotherapy. Researchers in Spain, Italy, and Japan have shown that melatonin guards against Adriamycin-induced damage to the heart, kidneys, brain, liver, bone marrow and lymphatic system. (290, 291, 293, 299, 368, 369) It also preserves blood levels of zinc in the body, which in turn aids in fighting the toxicity of the drug. (247)

Dr. Lissoni and his colleagues carried out a randomized clinical trial in 80 patients who had metastatic solid tumors and were in a poor clinical condition. Most of these had lung, breast, or gastrointestinal cancer. The lung cancer patients were treated with the standard drugs cisplatin and etoposide, breast cancer patients with mitoxantrone, and gastrointestinal tract tumor patients with 5-fluorouracil.

Patients were randomized to receive chemotherapy alone or chemotherapy plus melatonin. A type of white blood cell destruction (thrombocytopenia) was significantly less frequent in patients who also received melatonin. Malaise and weakness were also significantly less frequent in such patients.

Finally, mouth sores and nerve damage were less frequent in the melatonin group, although in this case the difference was not statistically significance. Hair loss and vomiting were not influenced by melatonin. They concluded that **"melatonin during chemotherapy may prevent some chemotherapy-induced side effects."** (243)

Another clinical trial was carried out to judge the effect of adding melatonin to the standard toxic drug epirubicin. Fourteen women with metastatic breast cancer women were given epirubicin weekly. Melatonin was also given orally, starting seven days prior to chemotherapy. Twelve patients could be evaluated after they received four cycles of chemotherapy.

Melatonin normalized the platelet count in 9 out of 12 of the women, and no further decline in clotting ability occurred in chemotherapy. Shrinkage of tumors was seen in 5 out of 12 (41 percent) of the women. "This study would suggest that melatonin may contribute to the realization of chemotherapy in metastatic cancer patients unable to tolerate the chemotherapeutic approach" because of persistent damage to the bone marrow. (236)

Dissenting Opinion

Unanimity is rare in science and scientific opinion is not unanimous on the value of using melatonin with chemotherapy. A small clinical trial in

Switzerland found no protective effect against the toxicity of carboplatin and etoposide in 20 patients with advanced lung cancer. The patients were given oral doses of melatonin at 40 milligrams per day for 21 days in the evening. Melatonin did not protect them against damage to the blood-forming system of carboplatin and etoposide. (133)

Melatonin and Leukemia—Caution?

There are concerns that melatonin—which powerfully boosts the immune system—might have a harmful effect in cancers of the immune system itself such as leukemia, lymphoma and myeloma. There is an animal experiment in which melatonin was shown to accelerate the growth of leukemia, while the surgical removal of the pineal gland (which produces melatonin) delayed it. (80a, 375) Because of this, I think it is best to err on the side of caution and not take melatonin if you have leukemia or other diseases characterized by the proliferation of white blood cells.

To summarize: The preponderance of laboratory and clinical data supports the use of melatonin in many kinds of cancer. Melatonin has its own anticancer effects, and also works well with cytokine therapy (interferon and interleukin) as well as with chemotherapy. But melatonin is not just an antioxidant, but a powerful hormone, and one must therefore be more cautious in its use in a self-help program.

The usual dosage in Dr. Lissoni's studies is 20 milligrams, taken a few hours before going to sleep. This is a large dose and I would suggest that you take this only under the guidance of a physician.

18. Folic Acid

Folic acid is one of the B vitamins that is crucial for the synthesis of DNA (genetic material) as well as for many other important cell functions. It was discovered in spinach leaves in 1941 and was named "folate," after the Latin word for leaf (*folium*). The terms folate and folic acid are roughly synonymous. For the sake of simplicity, I will generally use the latter term. Not surprisingly, this vitamin is mainly found in green leafy vegetables. Although folic acid is not an antioxidant, it boosts the antioxidant network and thus has a place in our story.

Folic Acid and Breast Cancer

Folic acid may reduce breast cancer risk, especially among women who drink alcoholic beverages. A study carried out at the Harvard School of Public Health examined the risk of breast cancer in 90,000 female nurses. Over the years, nearly 2,500 of them developed breast cancer. Folic acid consumption *per se* did not affect the rate of breast cancer.

However, in women who averaged one alcoholic drink per day, the risk of breast cancer was increased in those who also had the lowest folic acid intake. The risk of alcohol-associated breast cancer was reduced 45 percent in those who got the most folic acid.

"Our findings suggest that the excess risk of breast cancer associated with alcohol consumption may be reduced by adequate folate intake," the scientists concluded. (480)

The reader should note that there is a scientific controversy over whether or not alcohol consumption increases the risk of breast cancer. The latest findings do not show this, and in fact there are many other reasons to drink alcoholic beverages, especially red wine. However, women who do drink alcohol should make sure they also get an ample supply of folic acid in the form of green leafy vegetables and/or supplements.

Folic Acid, Alcohol and Colon Cancer

Some genetic mutations are actually beneficial. There is a mutation that about one-third of us have that is actually very favorable for preventing some common forms of cancer. Simply put, this mutation makes folic acid more readily available so that it can help with DNA repair.

In 1997, scientists at Harvard Medical School, Boston, looked for the effects of this beneficial genetic mutation in men with colon cancer. They also studied the same men for their alcohol intake. It turns out that having the desirable mutation while also drinking little or no alcohol has a remarkably protective effect.

Abstemious men had an **eight-fold decrease** in the risk of colon cancer. Moderate drinkers had a two-fold decrease in risk, but the advantage of the mutation disappears in men who have one or more drinks per day. This helps explain why low folic acid intake is associated with an increased risk of colon and rectal cancer. It also provides support for an important role of folic metabolism in the onset of colon and rectal cancer. (260)

Doctors do not regularly test for this mutation, although they might some day. For now, it is a good idea for all men to make sure they get an adequate intake of folic acid if they drink alcoholic beverages.

Folic Acid and Adult Leukemia

If you have this same mutated gene, you also have a much lower chance of getting acute lymphocytic leukemia (ALL) as an adult. The risk of ALL was reduced by two-thirds in those who had the mutated gene. Based on this finding, scientists at the University of California, Berkeley, have concluded that a lack of folic acid "may play a key role in the development of ALL" in adults. (414)

Folic Acid and Methotrexate

One of the firmest dogmas in cancer is that patients who are taking the chemotherapy drug methotrexate should not simultaneously take supplements of folic acid. Supposedly, the vitamin undoes the effects of the drug.

This position is mainly dictated by theory. However, there are hints in the literature that small doses of folic acid counteract the toxicity of methotrexate without impairing its effectiveness. Further research will be necessary to reach a conclusion.

Methotrexate was one of the first chemotherapeutic agents. More than 50 years ago, Dr. Sidney Farber of Boston tried to use folic acid as a treatment for leukemia. Instead of curing the children, however, it was his impression that folic acid actually accelerated the growth of the cancer. (157, 226) Farber then proceeded on the theory that if folic acid accelerates malignancies, an *antifolate* strategy might inhibit them.

First, he tried a folic acid-deprived diet, with some encouraging results. He then tested the first of the antifolate drugs, aminopterin, which was soon followed by methotrexate. (111) The results were historic, the first remissions in acute leukemia, which ushered in the so-called "Age of Miracles" of childhood cancer chemotherapy. (226) It also led to the growth of chemotherapy as an industry. One scientist has called methotrexate "an effective agent for treating cancer and building careers." (394)

Lower doses of methotrexate are now also used for certain non-malignant diseases, such as rheumatoid arthritis, acne, and psoriasis.

Methotrexate, Folic Acid and Arthritis

Methotrexate is sometimes used as a treatment for rheumatoid arthritis. Thirty-two arthritic patients were given folic acid supplements as well as methotrexate. This "significantly lowered toxicity scores without affecting efficacy. . . ." University of Alabama scientists wrote. (95, 296)

Similarly, Dutch scientists found that folic acid supplements had "no effect on the efficacy of methotrexate but may influence toxicity in a favorable way." (294) While no patients in the folic acid group discontinued methotrexate because of toxicity, four out of sixteen in the non-supplemented group did. (106, 333) An analysis of seven clinical trials showed that folic acid supplements led to a 79 percent reduction in side effects. (3) Admittedly, this is not cancer, and so we must be cautious in extrapolating from these results. But the results are provocative and suggest that reasonable doses of folic acid may protect against methotrexate toxicity and not interfere with its activity. This topic urgently deserves more clinical research.

Methotrexate causes an almost total deprivation of this vitamin—enough to kill the patient in high doses. Doctors sometimes deliberately give a deadly dose of methotrexate and then follow this with a synthetic form of folic acid called leucovorin. This rescue maneuver brings the patient back from the brink of death.

You can therefore understand the thinking of oncologists who for 50 years have warned patients never to take folic acid during methotrexate treatment. They are convinced that it might act as a kind of homemade rescue factor, competing successfully with the drug, and rendering its cell-killing activities null and void.

However, is it true that folic acid promotes the growth of existing cancers? No rigorous work has been done to evaluate the effects of folic acid supplements on the safety and effectiveness of methotrexate. Concerns are largely theoretical.

Typical of the confusion is an article on the topic at the peer-reviewed medical website, RxMED. It warns against the concurrent use of these two substances, saying "vitamin preparations containing folic acid or its derivatives may decrease responses to systemically administered methotrexate." A few paragraphs away, however, it states, "...large doses of folic acid given simultaneously will not reverse the effects of methotrexate." The webmasters never responded to my requests for clarification.

Danish researchers have found that children who were on a maintenance dose of methotrexate, and were also receiving folic acid supplements (75 to 200 micrograms) showed increased "hematological [blood] tolerance to methotrexate," as well as to a similar drug, 6-MP. This meant that they had higher counts of white blood cells than children who did not receive this supplement.

The scientists interpreted this to mean that a "proliferation" of white blood cells was undesirable and suggested that children in maintenance therapy not be given supplements containing folic acid. However, it is not specified whether the "proliferation" was of normal or malignant cells, and whether it was clinically harmful to these children. (396)

Lometrexal

Another study was done on a new anti-folic acid drug, Lometrexal. This drug had little toxicity in laboratory animals but severe toxicity in people. The reason turned out to be that lab animals routinely received folic acid supplements in their chow, whereas many people are deficient in the vitamin.

When scientists at the Eli Lilly company gave test animals, receiving Lometrexal, diets that were deficient in folic acid they reported that "remarkably, the lethality of this drug increased by three orders of magnitude in mildly folate-deficient mice." This "mimicked the unexpected toxicity seen in humans, they wrote. (225) The drug, which was not effective for breast cancer in folic acid-deficient mice, became so when it was given to supplemented animals.

But "excessively high folate intake reversed the antitumor effects" of the drug, as well. So they gave Lometrexal along with a *low dose* of folic acid. At such doses, the anticancer effects of Lometrexal in the body was "not altered by folic acid administration." (347)

Folic Acid and 5-FU

Folic acid works in tandem with another anticancer drug, 5-fluorouracil (or 5-FU). While 5-FU alone suppressed tumor growth 25 percent, adding folic acid increased growth suppression to over 70 percent. Scientists at the Medical College of South Carolina concluded, "These results indicate that folic acid is a potent modulator of 5-FU activity and could be considered as an alternative to leucovorin in the clinical setting."

To summarize: Although not itself an antioxidant, folic acid is an essential part of any anticancer program involving antioxidants. The data supporting the ban on folic acid for patients receiving methotrexate is surprisingly weak. However, for now it is probably wise to err on the side of caution and not take folic acid supplements if you are also taking methotrexate or other antifolate drugs.

19. History of a Controversy

You might wonder how scientists arrived at the idea that factors in food could protect us against cancer. Ever since cancer was first described —in the time of the Pharaohs—there have been theories linking the disease to dietary practices.

Some of these insights are particularly fascinating since they anticipate modern findings. Thus, the Roman author Cato advocated the crushed leaves of cabbage as a treatment for cancer, 2,000 years before the discovery that cruciferous vegetables, and especially cabbage, contain powerful anticancer elements. The famous ancient physician Galen worked out a comprehensive diet for cancer patients, which included poultry, vegetables, fish and red wine—all substances now known on scientific grounds to be beneficial to cancer patients.

When vitamins were discovered a century or so ago there was considerable interest in trying them out in cancer. In fact, until the emergence of chemotherapy, oncologists were receptive to this development. Speaking of these early attempts, the authors of a 1940 cancer textbook wrote, "Results have been impressive. In treating patients with incurable cancer, vitamins B and C seem to have a definite sphere for their administration, as well as vitamins A and D." (333)

Two-Edged Sword

Free radicals are a two-edged sword. While most are harmful, this is not necessarily so. They are also generated by our immune system to kill infectious organisms, as well as to eliminate abnormal cells. Thus, we don't want to get rid of all free radicals. But what we are seeking through the use of antioxidants is to harness and control them—to obtain their benefits without suffering too much from their harmful secondary effects.

The relationship of free radicals to health remained obscure for many years. In 1954, Denham Harman, then a graduate student at the University of California, Berkeley, proposed the "free radical theory of aging." He was largely ignored, although now this is considered a breakthrough moment in the history of nutritional science.

The increasing acceptance of Harman's theory in recent years has led inevitably to the question of cancer, since cancer is a disease that mainly strikes older people. The deeper scientists looked, the more evidence they found that cancer too was tied to free radical damage.

Today, free radical studies have blossomed in the scientific community. There are nearly 40,000 scientific articles on free radicals, and 50,000 on antioxidants, with more appearing daily. More than half of these have appeared in the last decade—a testimony to a quickening drumbeat of excitement. As Dr. Mitch Gaynor, M.D. and Jerry Hickey wrote in their excellent 1999 book, "No one knew the facts [about diet and cancer] until about ten years ago. In this relatively short span, the total weight of evidence has reached critical mass." (129)

Personal History

My own interest in cancer and nutrition began 25 years ago, when, as science writer for Memorial Sloan-Kettering Cancer Center in New York, I befriended Kanematsu Sugiura, D.Sc. Dr. Sugiura was one of the outstanding cancer scientists of the 20th century. (A picture of him at work at his bench graces the cover of Bristol-Myers Squibb's history of cancer research.) I had many teachers at Sloan-Kettering and am grateful to all of them. But Dr. Sugiura became my first mentor in the cancer field. Among other things, he introduced me to the work he did on nutrition and cancer just after World War One.

Some years later, I got to know Dr. Linus Pauling, the only man to win two unshared Nobel prizes. Dr. Pauling is best known for his advocacy of vitamin C, but he developed and named a new approach to healthcare called Orthomolecular Medicine (the use of substances that are natural to the human body.) Dr. Pauling's example as a scientist and a human being had a tremendous impact on me, as it did on thousands of other people.

But my most profound influence was Albert Szent-Györgyi, M.D., Ph.D., a scientist with whom I was closely associated for seven years, and whose biography I eventually wrote. Albert won the 1937 Nobel Prize for isolating and naming ascorbic acid (vitamin C). Among his other great discoveries were the bioflavonoids, which also figure in this story.

I called my biography of him *Free Radical*, not only because he himself was in every sense a "free radical," but because he was among the earliest to predict that the cancer problem would be solved at the level of electrons, which is where free radicals operate. I knew Albert when he was in his eighties and nineties, yet he was still hard at work every day on this electronic dimension of cancer. Incidentally, he attributed his longevity and health to liberal amounts of wheat germ and vitamin C.

One could not ask for better teachers than these. These great scientists collectively helped lay the groundwork for the current exciting work on antioxidants in the prevention and treatment of cancer. And each in his own way pointed me towards the topics you have read about in this book.

Changing Attitudes

In the last few years, we have witnessed a tremendous change in the attitude of scientists towards nutrition and cancer. For audiences of the 21st century, it will become increasingly difficult to understand how bitterly the American medical profession of the 20th century opposed the dietary approach to cancer. Doctors usually claimed they were defending the public from cancer quackery. But while there was some quackery, more often this charge was a figleaf to cover their fear of change.

Innovative doctors, who advocated a gentler, nutritional approach to cancer, were often ejected from their medical societies, set up for prosecution, driven out of the country, or even jailed. My book, *The Cancer Industry*, details many of their stories.

A low point came when the New York Medical Society took away the license of Max Gerson, M.D., a refugee from Nazism, who used a dietary approach to cancer. That diet was extremely high in fruits and vegetables. Gerson's sin was that he believed such a diet could not only prevent but treat advanced cancers.

In reference to his case, the *Journal of the American Medical Association* declared, in 1949, "There is no scientific evidence whatsoever to indicate that modifications in the dietary intake of food or other nutritional essentials are of any specific value in the control of cancer."

Fifty years later, in 1997, the same journal declared, **"The era of nutrient supplements to promote health and reduce illness is here to stay...There is overwhelming evidence of immunological enhancement following such an intervention."**

The same story could be told of many other pioneers, including an innovative dentist, William Donald Kelley, D.D.S., who advocated high-dose supplements and a dietary program, even for advanced pancreatic cancer. The U.S. government persecuted Kelley in the 1970s. Yet today, the NCI has committed over a million dollars to test the work of Nicholas Gonzalez, M.D., who follows the Kelley method.

There now is a committee at the National Institutes of Health whose sole purpose is to advise the government on alternative cancer treatments and an NCI office to coordinate its efforts. So things are changing.

What caused the cancer establishment to change?

Twenty-five years of struggle by thousands of individuals. Hundreds of popular books detailing advances in nutritional medicine. A broad international movement towards alternative medicine. And significant Congressional involvement. The conventional medical profession ignores such a broad movement at its own peril.

There are also thousands of scientific journal articles, from fine laboratories around the world, showing the beneficial effects of nutrients on serious problems such as heart disease and cancer.

Patients are increasingly becoming aware of this mountain of data. Doctors look foolish when their patients know more about nutrition than they do.

Then why, if you are a cancer patient, are you unlikely to have heard from your oncologist about using nutritional approaches?

Oncologists know toxic drugs, but are not trained in nutrition. They are intensely focused on surgery, radiation, and chemotherapy, but as a rule, they are not exposed to the latest advances in nutritional science. The medical journals that they read do not generally carry articles on the nutritional approach to cancer.

They are also unlikely to hear about these advances at their professional meetings. At the 1999 American Society of Clinical Oncology meeting in Atlanta, 2,500 studies were presented on various aspects of cancer treatment. And how many of these do you think were about antioxidants? Just one. (263)

Of the 1,800 clinical trials in the NCI database, how many involve treatment with antioxidants? It is hard to say, since there are no categories for antioxidants, vitamins, or nutritional therapies, to choose from. There may be a handful hidden away. But nutritional treatments are not being seriously investigated by many American oncologists.

Is it any wonder, then, that your own oncologist may be unaware of the positive developments in this field? For most of them, oncology means their own narrow discipline. **It is time for there to be a broader definition of oncology, one that incorporates nutritional treatments based on the latest scientific findings.**

Perhaps you will be one of those who opens your doctor's eyes to the enormous promise of using antioxidants in the fight against cancer.

20. *Conclusions*

Let me summarize the three basic ideas of this book:

- Antioxidants in fruits and vegetables reduce the risk of cancer.
- Supplements are a necessary part of any antioxidant program.
- Antioxidants generally improve conventional cancer treatments by decreasing side effects without decreasing effectiveness.

Dietary Antioxidants Protect Against Cancer

The data is very strong that eating a diet high in colorful fruits and vegetables strongly protects against cancers of many kinds. Fresh and frozen produce contain many antioxidants, other vitamins and minerals, and various interesting phytochemicals which prevent cancer from forming or progressing.

Any kind of colorful fruits and vegetables is preferable to none. However, I strongly recommend that you consume your produce either fresh or flash-frozen. I think that eating organic food makes a difference. You should patronize your health food store, organic market, and food coop.

During the summer, try to start a garden, which you can do even on a small patch of land, or a city terrace. Then freeze, or can, your excess for use in the non-summer months. Buy berries when they are abundant and freeze them.

The government recommends that you eat five half-cup servings of fruits and vegetables per day. Most adults get half this amount, and most children get one-quarter of their vegetable requirements.

Personally, I think you should reach higher…try to eat seven to ten half-cup portions per day. This means reorienting your diet, although it does not require strict vegetarianism.

Although all fruits and vegetables are important, you should put particular emphasis on berries, kale, garlic, tomatoes, and the other foods on the ORAC antioxidant list (see page 15).

Although the data is somewhat contradictory for women, I believe that moderate red wine usage is very healthful. Also try to drink three or four cups of tea each day.

Supplements Are a Part of Any Antioxidant Program

Taking food supplements can also help in the fight against cancer and many other health problems (such as heart disease).

If you are attempting to prevent the recurrence of cancer, you should probably be taking extra amounts of the supplements discussed in this book. Here is a program similar to what I and my family members take, although everyone's personal program has to be tailored to his or her individual circumstances:

1. A good multivitamin/mineral pill (without iron)
2. Vitamin A .... 10-20,000 IU
3. Vitamin C .... 500 to 2,000 milligrams
4. Vitamin E .... 200 to 1200 IU
5. Coenzyme Q10 .... 30 to 300 milligrams
6. Lipoic acid .... 50 to 200 milligrams
7. Zinc .... 15 to 30 milligrams
8. Selenium .... 200 micrograms
9. Pycnogenol, grape seeds .... 50 to 300 milligrams
10. Mixed carotenoids .... 10,000 to 25,000 IU

I strongly urge you to buy reputable national brands and to purchase natural (not synthetic) products. Supplements with iron should be avoided unless blood tests show you are anemic. As to vitamin E, you should alternate between mixed natural-source tocopherols and alpha-tocopherol succinate.

Antioxidants Help Conventional Cancer Treatments

I realize that the most controversial part of this book concerns my general recommendation that patients take antioxidants along with radiation and chemotherapy. However, the data overwhelmingly supports using antioxidants before, during, and after toxic treatments.

Consult a holistic doctor or nutritionist who can help you fine tune an antioxidant program for your particular needs.
This clinician can perform tests to make sure that the supplements you take are balancing your immune system.

I realize this advice flies in the face of many oncologists' opinions. While recognizing their theoretical concerns, I think we have to go where the data leads us: in this case the data is telling us that antioxidants have a beneficial effect on cancer patients.

Ten Cautionary Statements

There are some situations in which I think caution is advised. A few supplements may interact with particular forms of conventional therapy in a negative way. Most of these negative interactions have been found when single agents were tested, rather than a broad spectrum of nutrients, as listed above. Nevertheless, I have tried to make you aware of any "red flags" so that you can err on the side of caution.

Therefore, let me repeat the following cautionary statements on the use of specific supplements that I have discussed elsewhere in this book:

1. **Do not take very high doses of vitamins A, D or E, except under a doctor's direction.**
2. **Do not take synthetic beta-carotene, especially if you smoke.**
3. **Do not take high-dose vitamin C as a single agent while taking either methotrexate or DTIC.**
4. **Do not take high-dose vitamin C supplements if you have a hereditary tendency to accumulate iron (hemochromatosis).**
5. **Do not take NAC while you are taking cisplatin or Adriamycin.**
6. **Do not take high-dose tangeretin, especially with tamoxifen.**
7. **Do not take zinc while you are taking cisplatin or carboplatin.**
8. **Do not take melatonin if you have leukemia or any other proliferative disease of the blood or lymph.**
9. **Do not take folic acid while you are taking methotrexate.**
10. **Have your progress checked by a holistic clinician.**

Secrecy

Nor am I suggesting that you take antioxidants or other supplements behind the back of your oncologists. Surveys show that many people are doing precisely that. (373) I think it is unwise. Your doctor is a key member of your team and needs to know what other treatments you are doing.

Secrecy can backfire in unexpected way. For instance, I have heard of cases in which oncologists increased their patients' doses when they did not have the expected side effects of chemotherapy!

If you feel the need to be less than forthright with your oncologist, this indicates a serious problem in communications. Have you taken steps to correct this? For instance, try writing down your questions before you go for your office visit, and make sure you take an advocate with you to take notes and bring up relevant points. If your oncologist rushes you, or is dismissive of your concerns, you may have to look for another doctor.

The best thing is to respectfully inform them of your wishes to take antioxidants alongside conventional treatment. If they are resistant, try to reason with them. A copy of this book given as a gift may be able to change their minds.

If your doctor is adamantly opposed, you might try taking supplements *before* and *after* conventional treatment, while foregoing them during conventional therapy itself. This may not be as effective at curbing side effects, but will still be beneficial. In the end, though, both legally and morally, *it is your body and your choice*. The oncologist is there to serve you, and not the other way around. My wishes are with you to choose wisely.

The Antioxidant Revolution

As I wrote this book I became increasingly excited about the prospects of using antioxidants and other nutrients to prevent and treat cancer.

Although I listened to radio nutritionist Dr. Carlton Fredericks on my mother's knee, and started taking vitamins after reading Adelle Davis, I have now redoubled my efforts. I eat lots of organic fruits and vegetables and take almost all of the major antioxidants on a daily basis.

It is hard to avoid clichés when writing about this topic. Words like "miracle" and "revolution" flow too easily off the tongue. But I think in the case of antioxidants and nutritional medicine they are justified. The turn towards nutritional therapies has the feeling of something big, a long-awaited turn towards a new kind of healthcare, compared to which conventional medicine will seem like medieval barbarity.

There have always been pioneers who have advocated the nutritional approach to cancer. They were dismissed as irrational, or worse, but now we understand the scientific basis for many of their beliefs. I foresee the day when *all* doctors will be trained in the use of food and food supplements to fight cancer. But you needn't wait for that glorious day.

You can take part in this Antioxidant Revolution now. Increase your daily intake of antioxidants and share your program with friends, relatives, neighbors, and especially doctors. In this way, you will not only help yourself but will accelerate the pace of change.

By fostering this movement, you hasten the day that antioxidants will no longer be the stepchild of oncology, but the first thing doctors and patients turn to in the fight against cancer.

Appendix: Synthetic Antioxidants

There is a class of prescription drugs whose existence strongly supports my argument about the benefit of dietary antioxidants for cancer patients on radiation and chemotherapy. These are the synthetic antioxidants. They were created in chemistry labs to mimic (and presumably improve upon) the effects of dietary antioxidants. These agents are now routinely used by oncologists around the world to lessen the severity of radiation and toxic chemotherapy.

All have been extensively investigated in the laboratory and the clinic and all have been found relatively safe and effective. They are approved by governmental agencies, such as the FDA. In other words, they are not the subject of controversy. No oncologists worry that they will interfere with radiation or chemotherapy. In fact, they use them precisely as I suggest using natural antioxidants, to reduce the side effects of conventional treatment. The use of these synthetic agents shows that antioxidants in general are unlikely to harm cancer patients.

The following is a brief discussion of the three most common synthetic antioxidants:

Amifostine (WR-2721)

Amifostine is a synthetic variant on the amino acid cysteine. In 1949, a doctor noted that cysteine protects animals from the side effects of radiation. (344) Under the auspices of the U.S. Army, Amifostine (also called WR-2721) was created. The first clinical trial was carried out in the 1970s in Japan and showed a beneficial effect on patients receiving radiation therapy. (437) Five out of thirty-seven rectal cancer patients who received radiation treatment without amifostine had moderate-to-severe side effects. But of 34 patients who got amifostine, none had such side effects. The complete response rate to treatment was also higher (16 versus 10 percent). (207)

Unfortunately, this synthetic drug has considerable toxicity of its own when administered with radiation therapy and is therefore inferior to the natural antioxidants described in this book.

Amifostine "reduced radiation-induced toxicities without reducing antitumor efficacy," said doctors at the University of Wisconsin Medical School. (274) A major radiation textbook concurs: "No evidence of tumor protection from WR-2721 has been observed in these clinical studies." (345) ("Tumor protection" refers to a drug's ability to shield the cancer itself from the effects of treatment.) These findings should calm the fear of oncologists that antioxidants interfere with radiation treatments.

Mesna

Mesna is a synthetic antioxidant that protects against the dangerous side effects of the drug ifosfamide (Ifex). Ifosfamide can damage the urinary system by causing hemorrhagic cystitis (blood in the urine). Mesna unites with a harmful substance to form a non-toxic compound that is then eliminated in the urine. (49) Mesna emerged from a nonconventional cancer clinic, but is now accepted around the world. It is not necessary to cite dozens of studies showing that mesna is a safe and effective adjunct to ifosfamide. So here's another instance in which a powerful antioxidant not only does not interfere with chemotherapy but is routinely used alongside it by all oncologists who use ifosfamide.

ICRF-187 (dexrazoxane or Cardiozane)

ICRF-187 (also called dexrazoxane or Cardiozane) is another synthetic antioxidant. It is widely used to counteract Adriamycin's toxicity. There are over 500 papers on this drug, and they show that it is a reasonably effective heart protector. (7, 8, 161-164, 486) This statement is not controversial, and ICRF-187 is universally accepted for this purpose.

To give one example out of many: in a clinical trial, the drug epirubicin (similar in structure to Adriamycin) damaged the hearts of about a quarter of the patients who took it. But when patients were given ICRF-187, only 7.3 percent of patients were injured. The rates of tumor shrinkage, of progression-free survival, and of overall survival were similar in both groups. Adding this powerful synthetic antioxidant did not undermine the clinical activity of chemotherapy. It only helped the patients. (458)

To summarize: oncologists routinely prescribe synthetic antioxidants along with radiation and chemotherapy.

It is an uncontested fact that synthetic antioxidants do not have a negative impact on radiation and chemotherapy treatments, nor do oncologists fear that they might. **Instead, synthetic antioxidants preserve the effectiveness of conventional treatments while reducing their harmful side effects.** The data also supports the idea that dietary antioxidants protect against harmful side effects, without interfering with the cancer-killing ability of conventional treatments. And natural antioxidants do this without toxic side effects of their own and at a fraction of the cost of these synthetic agents.

Further Reading: A Short List

Atkins, Robert, *Dr. Atkins' Vita-Nutrient Solution.* New York, NY: Simon and Schuster, 1999. An inspiring work based on 30 years experience.

Boik, John, *Cancer and Natural Medicine*. Princeton, MN.: Oregon Medical Press, 1996. A very scholarly work, cautious but informative.

Gaynor, Mitch and Jerry Hickey, *Dr. Gaynor's Cancer Prevention Program.* New York, NY: Kensington, 1999. An open-minded oncologist and a holistic pharmacist team up to create an excellent program.

Goodman, Sandra. *Nutrition and Cancer: State of the Art.* Bristol, England: Positive Health Publications, 1998. An excellent summary from Britain of the scientific data on antioxidants and other nutrients.

Hendler, Sheldon Saul. *The Doctor's Vitamin and Mineral Encyclopedia.* New York: Simon & Schuster, 1990. A comprehensive guide.

Moss, Ralph W. *Cancer Therapy.* Brooklyn, NY: Equinox, 2nd Ed., 1996. In this work, I present the scientific evidence for the validity of 102 different non-conventional cancer treatments, including vitamins.

Packer, Lester and Carol Coleman, *The Antioxidant Miracle.* New York, NY: Wiley, 1999. A really fine overview of the field from "Dr. Antioxidant."

Passwater, Richard A., *Cancer Prevention and Nutritional Therapies.* New Canaan, CT: Keats, 1983. One of the original and still excellent works.

Prasad, Kedar, *Vitamins in Cancer Prevention and Treatment.* Rochester, VT: Inner Traditions International Ltd., 1993. Sensible advice from one of the true pioneers of antioxidant research in the United States. Excellent.

Quillin, Patrick, *Beating Cancer with Nutrition.* Tulsa, OK: Nutrition Times Press, 1998. An upbeat, fact-filled and inspiring presentation from the nutrition director of a large cancer center.

Simone, Charles, *Cancer and Nutrition.* Garden City Park, NY: Avery Publishing Group, 1992. A groundbreaking guide from an oncologist, very strong on the advisability of using antioxidants with chemotherapy.

References

1. Agarwal, S., and Rao A.V. Tomato lycopene and low-density lipoprotein oxidation: a human dietary intervention study. Lipids 1998;33:981-984.
2. Agus DB, et al. Stromal cell oxidation: a mechanism by which tumors obtain vitamin C. Cancer Res. 1999 Sep 15;59(18):4555-8.
3. Alati T, et al. Augmentation of the therapeutic activity of lometrexol -(6-R)5,10-dideazatetrahydrofolate- by oral folic acid. Cancer Res. 1996 May 15;56(10):2331-5.
4. Albanes D, et al. Alpha-Tocopherol and beta-carotene supplements and lung cancer incidence in the alpha-tocopherol, beta-carotene cancer prevention study: effects of base-line characteristics and study compliance. J Natl Cancer Inst. 1996 Nov 6;88(21):1560-70.
5. Alberts DS, et al. alpha-Tocopherol pretreatment increases adriamycin bone marrow toxicity. Biomedicine. 1978 Oct;29(6):189-91.
6. Albini A, et al. Inhibition of invasion, gelatinase activity, tumor take and metastasis of malignant cells by N-acetylcysteine. Int J Cancer. 1995 Mar 29;61(1):121-9.
7. Alderton P, et al. Role of (+-)-1,2-bis(3,5-dioxopiperazinyl-1-yl)propane (ICRF-187) in modulating free radical scavenging enzymes in doxorubicin-induced cardiomyopathy. Cancer Res. 1990 Aug 15;50(16):5136-42.
8. Alderton PM, et al. Comparative study of doxorubicin, mitoxantrone, and epirubicin in combination with ICRF-187 (ADR-529) in a chronic cardiotoxicity animal model. Cancer Res. 1992 Jan 1;52(1):194-201.
9. Allen, C, et al. Bed rest: a potentially harmful treatment needing more careful evaluation. Lancet 1999;354:1229.
10. Amara-Mokrane YA, et al. Protective effects of alpha-hederin, chlorophyllin and ascorbic acid towards the induction of micronuclei by doxorubicin in cultured human lymphocytes. Mutagenesis [formation of mutations]. 1996 Mar;11(2):161-7.
11. Ames BN. Micronutrients prevent cancer and delay aging. Toxicol Lett. 1998 Dec 28;102-103:5-18.
12. Anderson PM, et al. Oral glutamine reduces the duration and severity of stomatitis after cytotoxic cancer chemotherapy. Cancer. 1998 Oct 1;83(7):1433-9.
13. Andrieu-Abadie N, et al. L-carnitine prevents doxorubicin-induced apoptosis of cardiac myocytes: role of inhibition of ceramide generation. FASEB J. 1999 Sep;13(12):1501-1510.
14. Andriole GL, et al. The efficacy of mesna (2-mercaptoethane sodium sulfonate) as a uroprotectant in patients with hemorrhagic cystitis receiving further oxazaphosphorine chemotherapy. J Clin Oncol. 1987 May;5(5):799-803.
15. Anon., The alpha-tocopherol, beta-carotene lung cancer prevention study: design, methods, participant characteristics, and compliance. The ATBC Cancer Prevention Study Group. Ann Epidemiol 1994 Jan;4(1):1-10.
16. Antunes LM, et al. Effects of high doses of vitamins C and E against doxorubicin-induced chromosomal damage in Wistar rat bone marrow cells. Mutat Res. 1998 Nov 9;419(1-3):137-43.
17. Antunes LM, et al. Protection and induction of chromosomal damage by vitamin C in human lymphocyte cultures. Teratog Carcinog Mutagen. 1999;19(1):53-9.
18. Appenroth D, et al. Protective effects of vitamin E and C on cisplatin nephrotoxicity in developing rats. Arch Toxicol. 1997;71(11):677-83.
19. Atkins, Robert, Dr. Atkins' Vita-Nutrient Solution, New York, NY 1999.
20. Atukorala TM, et al. Longitudinal studies of nutritional status in patients having chemotherapy for testicular teratomas. Clin Oncol. 1983 Mar;9(1):3-10. Auer BL, et al. Relative hyperoxaluria, crystalluria and haematuria after megadose ingestion of vitamin C. Eur J Clin Invest. 1998 Sep;28(9):695-700.
21. Auer BL, et al. The effect of ascorbic acid ingestion on the biochemical and physicochemical risk factors associated with calcium oxalate kidney stone formation. Clin Chem Lab Med. 1998 Mar;36(3):143-7.
22. Badylak SF, et al. Poikilocytosis in dogs with chronic doxorubicin toxicosis. Am J Vet Res. 1985 Feb;46(2):505-8.
23. Banic S. Vitamin C acts as a cocarcinogen to methylcholanthrene in guinea-pigs. Cancer Lett. 1981 Jan;11(3):239-42.
24. Barbone F, et al. A Follow-up Study of Determinants of Second Tumor and Metastasis Among Subjects with Cancer of the Oral Cavity, Pharynx and Larynx. J Clin Epidemiol 1996;49:367-372.
25. Barni S, et al. A randomized study of low-dose subcutaneous interleukin-2 plus melatonin versus supportive care alone in metastatic colorectal cancer patients progressing under 5-fluorouracil and folates. Oncology. 1995 May-Jun;52(3):243-5.
26. Bartlett DL, et al. Effect of glutamine on tumor and host growth. Ann Surg Oncol. 1995 Jan;2(1):71-6.
27. Batieha AM, et al. Serum Micronutrients and the Subsequent Risk of Cervical Cancer in a Population- Based Nested Case-Control Study. Cancer Epid Biomarkers Prev 1993;2:335-339.
28. Battelli D, et al. Interaction of carnitine with mitochondrial cardiolipin. Biochim Biophys Acta. 1992 Jul 21;1117(1):33-6.
29. Ben-Amotz A, et al. Bioavailability of a natural isomer mixture as compared with synthetic all-trans-beta-carotene in rats and chicks. J Nutr. 1989 Jul;119(7):1013-9.
30. Benedict WF, et al. Differences in anchorage-dependent growth and tumorigenicities between transformed C3H/10T 1/2 cells with morphologies that are or are not reverted to a normal phenotype by ascorbic acid. Cancer Res. 1982 Mar;42(3):1041-5.
31. Benner SE, et al. Regression of oral leukoplakia with alpha-tocopherol: a community clinical oncology program chemoprevention study. J Natl Cancer Inst. 1993 Jan 6;85(1):44-7.
32. Berger M, et al. [Effect of thioctic acid (alpha-lipoic acid) on the chemotherapeutic efficacy of cyclophosphamide and vincristine sulfate]. Arzneimittelforschung. 1983;33(9):1286-8.

33. Bertazzoli C, et al. Adriamycin associated cardiotoxicity: research on prevention with coenzyme Q. Pharmacol Res Commun. 1977 Mar;9(3):235-50.

34. Bertazzoli C, et al. Effect of Adriamycin on the activity of the succinate dehydrogenase-coenzyme Q10 reductase of the rabbit myocardium. Res Commun Chem Pathol Pharmacol. 1976 Dec;15(4):797-800.

35. Besa EC, et al. A pilot trial of 13-cis-retinoic acid and alpha-tocopherol with recombinant human erythropoietin in myelodysplastic syndrome patients with progressive or transfusion-dependent anemias. The Central Pennsylvania Oncology Group. Leuk Res. 1998 Aug;22(8):741-9.

36. Bjelke, E. Dietary factors and the epidemiology of cancer of the stomach and large bowel. Aktuel Ernaehrungsmed Klin Prax Suppl 1978;2:10-17.

37. Bjelke, E. Dietary vitamin A and human lung cancer. Int J Cancer 1975;15:561-565.

38. Bliznakov EG. Immunological senescence in mice and its reversal by coenzyme Q10. Mech Ageing Dev. 1978 Mar;7(3):189-97.

39. Blomgren H, et al. Antitumor activity of 2-mercaptoethanesulfonate (mesna) in vitro. Its potential use in the treatment of superficial bladder cancer. Anticancer Res. 1991 Mar-Apr;11(2):773-6.

40. Blomgren H, et al. Antitumor activity of 2-mercaptoethanesulfonate (mesna) in vitro. Methods Find Exp Clin Pharmacol. 1990 Dec;12(10):691-7.

41. Blomgren H, et al. Inhibition of tumor cell growth in vitro by 2-mercaptoethanesulfonate (mesna) and other thiols. Methods Find Exp Clin Pharmacol. 1991 Oct;13(8):579-82.

42. Bogin E, et al. Changes in serum, liver and kidneys of cisplatin-treated rats; effects of antioxidants. Eur J Clin Chem Clin Biochem. 1994 Nov;32(11):843-51.

43. Bohlke K, et al. Vitamins A, C and E and the risk of breast cancer: results from a case-control study in Greece. Br J Cancer. 1999 Jan;79(1):23-9.

44. Bomser J, et al. In vitro anticancer activity of fruit extracts from Vaccinium species. Planta Med. 1996 Jun;62(3):212-6.

45. Boscoboinik D, et al. Alpha-tocopherol (vitamin E) regulates vascular smooth muscle cell proliferation and protein kinase C activity. Arch Biochem Biophys. 1991 Apr;286(1):264-9.

46. Bracke ME, et al. Influence of tangeretin on tamoxifen's therapeutic benefit in mammary cancer. J Natl Cancer Inst. 1999 Feb 17;91(4):354-9.

47. Bram S, et al. Vitamin C preferential toxicity for malignant melanoma cells. Nature. 1980 Apr 17;284(5757):629-31.

48. Breed JG, et al.Failure of the antioxidant vitamin E to protect against adriamycin-induced cardiotoxicity in the rabbit. Cancer Res. 1980 Jun;40(6):2033-8.

49. Brock N, et al. Acrolein, the causative factor of urotoxic side-effects of cyclophosphamide, ifosfamide, trofosfamide and sufosfamide. Arzneimittelforschung. 1979;29(4):659-61.

50. Brotzman, M, et al. Vitamin supplement use and p53 mutations in head and neck cancer. Proc AACR, Abstract #4126, March, 1999.

51. Burke KE, et al. The effects of topical and oral L-selenomethionine on pigmentation and skin cancer induced by ultraviolet irradiation. Nutr Cancer 1992;17(2):123-37.

52. Busse E, et al. Influence of alpha-lipoic acid on intracellular glutathione in vitro and in vivo. Arzneimittelforschung. 1992 Jun;42(6):829-31.

53. Bussey HJ, et al. A randomized trial of ascorbic acid in polyposis coli. Cancer 1982;50:1434-1439.

54. Caffrey PB, et al. Prevention of the development of melphalan resistance in vitro by selenite. Biol Trace Elem Res. 1998 Dec;65(3):187-95.

55. Caffrey PB, et al. Sensitivity of melphalan-resistant tumors to selenite in vivo. Cancer Lett. 1997 Dec 23;121(2):177-80.

56. Caffrey PB, et al. Treatment of human ovarian tumor xenografts with selenite prevents the melphalan-induced development of drug resistance. Anticancer Res. 1998 Jul-Aug;18(4C):3017-20.

57. Cai L, et al. Protective role of zinc-metallothionein on DNA damage in vitro by ferric nitrilotriacetate (Fe-NTA) and ferric salts. Chem Biol Interact. 1998 Sep 4;115(2):141-51.

58. Cameron E, et al. Innovation vs. quality control: an 'unpublishable' clinical trial of supplemental ascorbate in incurable cancer. Med Hypotheses. 1991 Nov;36(3):185-9.

59. Cao, G, et al. Oxygen-radical absorbance capacity assay for antioxidants. Free Radic Biol Med. 1993 Mar;14(3):303-11.

60. Capel ID, et al. Vitamin E retards the lipoperoxidation resulting from anticancer drug administration. Anticancer Res. 1983 Jan-Feb;3(1):59-62.

61. Carr A, et al. Does vitamin C act as a pro-oxidant under physiological conditions? FASEB J. 1999 Jun;13(9):1007-24.

62. Carr AC, et al.Toward a new recommended dietary allowance for vitamin C based on antioxidant and health effects in humans. Am J Clin Nutr. 1999 Jun;69(6):1086-107.

63. Cheshier JE, et al. Immunomodulation by pycnogenol in retrovirus-infected or ethanol-fed mice. Life Sci. 1996;58(5):PL 87-96.

64. Chida M, et al. In vitro testing of antioxidants and biochemical end-points in bovine retinal tissue. Ophthalmic Res. 1999 Nov;31(6):407-415.

65. Chinery R, et al. Antioxidants enhance the cytotoxicity of chemotherapeutic agents in colorectal cancer: a p53-independent induction of p21WAF1/CIP1 via C/EBPbeta. Nat Med. 1997 Nov;3(11):1233-41.

66. Choe JY, et al. Prevention by coenzyme Q10 of the electrocardiographic changes induced by Adriamycin in rats. Res Commun Chem Pathol Pharmacol. 1979 Jan;23(1):199-202.

67. Choe JY, et al. Study of the combined and separate administration of doxorubicin and coenzyme Q10 on mouse cardiac enzymes. Res Commun Chem Pathol Pharmacol. 1979 Jun;24(3):595-8.

68. Chopra RK, et al. Relative bioavailability of coenzyme Q10 formulations in human subjects. Int J Vitam Nutr Res. 1998;68(2):109-13.

69. Ciaccio M, et al. Vitamin A preserves the cytotoxic activity of adriamycin while counteracting its peroxidative effects in human leukemic cells in vitro. Biochem Mol Biol Int. 1994 Sep;34(2):329-35.

70. Clark LC, et al. Decreased incidence of prostate cancer with selenium supplementation: results of a double-blind cancer prevention trial. Br J Urol. 1998 May;81(5):730-4.

71. Clark LC, et al. Effects of selenium supplementation for cancer prevention in patients with car-

cinoma of the skin. A randomized controlled trial. Nutritional Prevention of Cancer Study Group. JAMA. 1996 Dec 25;276(24):1957-63.

72. Clemens MR, et al. Decreased essential antioxidants and increased lipid hydroperoxides following high-dose radiochemotherapy. Free Radic Res Commun. 1989;7(3-6):227-32.

73. Clemens MR, et al. Plasma vitamin E and beta-carotene concentrations during radiochemotherapy preceding bone marrow transplantation. Am J Clin Nutr. 1990 Feb;51(2):216-9.

74. Clemens MR, et al. Supplementation with antioxidants prior to bone marrow transplantation. Wien Klin Wochenschr. 1997 Oct 17;109(19):771-6.

75. Cohen M, et al. Ascorbic acid and gastrointestinal cancer. J Am Coll Nutr. 1995 Dec;14(6): 565-78.

76. Combs AB, et al. Models for clinical disease. I. Biochemical cardiotoxicity of a coenzyme Q10-inhibitor in rats. Res Commun Chem Pathol Pharmacol. 1976 Feb;13(2):333-9.

77. Combs AB, et al. Reduction by coenzyme Q10 of the acute toxicity of Adriamycin in mice. Res Commun Chem Pathol Pharmacol. 1977 Nov;18(3):565-8.

78. Combs GF Jr, et al. Reduction of cancer risk with an oral supplement of selenium. Biomed Environ Sci. 1997 Sep;10(2-3):227-34.

79. Connors, TA. Mechanisms of clinical drug resistance. Biochem Pharm 1974;23 (suppl. 2) 89-100.

80. Conte A, et al. Synergic and complementary effects of L-carnitine and coenzyme Q on long-chain fatty acid metabolism and on protection against anthracycline damage. Int J Tissue React. 1990;12(3):197-201.

81. Conti A', Role of pineal melatonin and melatonin-induced-immuno-opioids in murine leukemogenesis. Med Oncol Tumor Pharmacother. 1992;9(2):87-92.

81. Cook-Mozaffari PJ, et al. Oesophageal cancer studies in the Caspian Littoral of Iran: results of a case-control study. Br J Cancer. 1979 Mar;39(3):293-309.

82. Cooke MS, et al. Novel repair action of vitamin C upon in vivo oxidative DNA damage. FEBS Lett. 1998 Nov 20;439(3):363-7.

83. Cortes EP, et al. Adriamycin cardiotoxicity: early detection by systolic time interval and possible prevention by coenzyme Q10. Cancer Treat Rep. 1978 Jun;62(6):887-91.

84. Cossins E, et al. ESR studies of vitamin C regeneration, order of reactivity of natural source phytochemical preparations. Biochem Mol Biol Int. 1998 Jul;45(3):583-97.

85. Dartigues J, et al. Dietary vitamin A, beta-carotene and risk of epidermoid lung cancer in southwestern France. European Journal of Epidemiology 1990;6:261-65.

86. De Flora S, et al. Synergism between N-acetylcysteine and doxorubicin in the prevention of tumorigenicity and metastasis in murine models. Int J Cancer. 1996 Sep 17;67(6):842-8.

87. De Leonardis V, et al. Reduction of cardiac toxicity of anthracyclines by L-carnitine: preliminary overview of clinical data. Int J Clin Pharmacol Res. 1985;5(2):137-42.

88. De Loecker W, et al. Effects of sodium ascorbate (vitamin C) and 2-methyl-1,4-naphthoquinone (vitamin K3) treatment on human tumor cell growth in vitro. II. Synergism with combined chemotherapy action. Anticancer Res. 1993 Jan-Feb;13(1):103-6.

89. Decker-Baumann C, et al. Reduction of chemotherapy-induced side-effects by parenteral glutamine supplementation in patients with metastatic colorectal cancer. Eur J Cancer. 1999 Feb;35(2):202-7.

90. DeCosse, JJ, et al. Effect of ascorbic acid on rectal polyps of patients with familial polyposis. Surgery 1975;78:608-612.

91. De Vries N and Snow G. Relationship of vitamins A and E and beta-carotene serum levels to head and neck cancer patients with and without second primary tumors. European Archies of Otolaryngol 1990;247:368-70.

92. Di Re F, et al. Efficacy and safety of high-dose cisplatin and cyclophosphamide with glutathione protection in the treatment of bulky advanced epithelial ovarian cancer. Cancer Chemother Pharmacol. 1990;25(5):355-60.

93. Di Re F, et al. High-dose cisplatin and cyclophosphamide with glutathione in the treatment of advanced ovarian cancer. Ann Oncol. 1993 Jan;4(1):55-61.

94. Diplock AT. Will the 'good fairies' please prove to us that vitamin E lessens human degenerative disease? Free Radic Res. 1997 Nov;27(5):511-32.

95. Dijkmans BA. Folate supplementation and methotrexate. Br J Rheumatol. 1995 Dec;34(12):1172-4

96. Dimery IW, et al. Phase I trial of alpha-tocopherol effects on 13-cis-retinoic acid toxicity. Ann Oncol. 1997 Jan;8(1):85-9.

97. Donaldson SS, et al. Alterations of nutritional status: impact of chemotherapy and radiation therapy. Cancer. 1979 May;43(5 Suppl):2036-52.

98. Dorr RT. Cytoprotective agents for anthracyclines. Semin Oncol. 1996 Aug;23(4 Suppl 8):23-34.

99. Doz F, et al. Metallothionein and anticancer agents: the role of metallothionein in cancer chemotherapy. J Neurooncol. 1993 Aug;17(2):123-9.

100. Doz F et al., Experimental basis for increasing the therapeutic index of cis-diamminedicarboxylatocyclobutaneplatinum(II) in brain tumor therapy by a high-zinc diet. Cancer Chemother Pharmacol 1992;29:219-26.

101. Drago JR, et al. Chemotherapy and vitamin E in treatment of Nb rat prostate tumors. In Vivo. 1988 Nov-Dec;2(6):399-401.

102. el Daly ES. Protective effect of cysteine and vitamin E, Crocus sativus and Nigella sativa extracts on cisplatin-induced toxicity in rats. J Pharm Belg. 1998 Mar-Apr;53(2):87-93.

103. Eichholzer M, et al. Smoking, plasma vitamins C, E, retinol, and carotene, and fatal prostate cancer: seventeen-year follow-up of the prospective Basel study. Prostate. 1999 Feb 15;38(3):189-98.

104. el-Nahas SM, et al. Radioprotective effect of vitamins C and E. Mutat Res. 1993 Feb;301(2):143-7.

105. Elgohary WG, et al. Protection of DNA in HL-60 cells from damage generated by hydroxyl radicals produced by reaction of H2O2 with cell iron by zinc-metallothionein. Chem Biol Interact. 1998 Sep 4;115(2):85-107.

106. Endresen GK, et al. [Methotrexate and folates in rheumatoid arthritis]. Tidsskr Nor Laegeforen. 1999 Feb 10;119(4):534-7.

107. Epstein JH. Effects of beta-carotene on ultraviolet induced cancer formation in the hairless mouse skin. Photochem Photobiol. 1977 Feb;25(2):211-3.

108. Erhola, M ,et al. Effect of anthracycline-based chemotherapy on total plasma antioxidant capacity in small-cell lung cancer patients. Free Radic Biol Med 1996;21:383-390.

109. Evangelou A, et al. Dose-related preventive and therapeutic effects of antioxidants-anticarcinogens on experimentally induced malignant tumors in Wistar rats. Cancer Lett. 1997 May 1;115(1):105-11.

110. Evans WK, et al. A randomized study of oral nutritional support versus ad lib nutritional intake during chemotherapy for advanced colorectal and non-small-cell lung cancer. J Clin Oncol. 1987 Jan;5(1):113-24.

111. Farber, S, et al. Temporary remissions in acute leukemia in children produced by folic acid antagonist, 4-aminopteroyl-glutamic acid (aminopterin). N Engl J Med 1948;238:787.

112. Faure H, et al. [Carotenoids: 2. Diseases and supplementation studies]. Ann Biol Clin (Paris). 1999 May;57(3):273-82.

112a. Feldman D, et al. Vitamin D and prostate cancer. Adv Exp Med Biol. 1995;375:53-63.

113. Felemovicius I, et al. Intestinal radioprotection by vitamin E (alpha-tocopherol). Ann Surg. 1995 Oct;222(4):504-8; discussion 508-10.

115. Floersheim GL, et al. Radiation-induced lymphoid tumors and radiation lethality are inhibited by combined treatment with small doses of zinc aspartate and WR 2721. Int J Cancer. 1992 Oct 21;52(4):604-8.

116. Folkers K, et al. The activities of coenzyme Q10 and vitamin B6 for immune responses. Biochem Biophys Res Commun. 1993 May 28;193(1): 88-92.

117. Folkers K, et al. Activities of vitamin Q10 in animal models and a serious deficiency in patients with cancer. Biochem Biophys Res Commun. 1997 May 19;234(2):296-9.

118. Folkers K, et al. Inhibition by Adriamycin of the mitochondrial biosynthesis of coenzyme Q10 and implication for the cardiotoxicity of Adriamycin in cancer patients. Biochem Biophys Res Commun. 1977 Aug 22;77(4):1536-42.

119. Folkers K, et al. Rescue by coenzyme Q10 from electrocardiographic abnormalities caused by the toxicity of Adriamycin in the rat. Proc Natl Acad Sci U S A. 1978 Oct;75(10):5178-80.

120. Folkers K, et al. Research on coenzyme Q10 in clinical medicine and in immunomodulation. Drugs Exp Clin Res. 1985;11(8):539-45.

121. Folkers K, et al. Survival of cancer patients on therapy with coenzyme Q10. Biochem Biophys Res Commun. 1993 Apr 15;192(1):241-5.

122. Franceschi S, et al. Tomatoes and risk of digestive tract cancers. Int J Cancer 1994;59:181-184.

123. Freudenheim JL, et al. Premenopausal breast cancer risk and intake of vegetables, fruits, and related nutrients. J Natl Cancer Inst. 1996 Mar 20;88(6):340-8.

124. Fujita K, et al. Reduction of adriamycin toxicity by ascorbate in mice and guinea pigs. Cancer Res. 1982 Jan;42(1):309-16.

125. Funegard U, et al. Can alpha-tocopherol and beta-carotene supplementation reduce adverse radiation effects on salivary glands? Eur J Cancer. 1995 Dec;31A(13-14):2347-53.

126. Gardiner NS, et al. Enhanced prostaglandin synthesis as a mechanism for inhibition of melanoma cell growth by ascorbic acid. Prostaglandins Leukot Essent Fatty Acids. 1988 Nov;34(2):119-26.

127. Gardiner NS, et al. Inhibition of murine melanoma growth by sodium ascorbate. J Nutr. 1989 Apr;119(4):586-90.

128. Gartner C, et al. Lycopene is more bioavailable from tomato paste than from fresh tomatoes. Am J Clin Nutr. 1997 Jul;66(1):116-22.

129. Gaynor, M and Hickey J. Dr. Gaynor's Cancer Prevention Program. .New York: Kensington, 1999.

130. Geetha A, et al. Effect of alpha-tocopherol on peroxidative membrane damage caused by doxorubicin: an in vitro study in human erythrocytes. Indian J Exp Biol. 1989 Mar;27(3):274-8.

131. German JB. Food processing and lipid oxidation.Adv Exp Med Biol 1999;459:23-50

132. Gerster H. High-dose vitamin C: a risk for persons with high iron stores? Int J Vitam Nutr Res. 1999 Mar;69(2):67-82

133. Ghielmini M, et al. Double-blind randomized study on the myeloprotective effect of melatonin in combination with carboplatin and etoposide in advanced lung cancer. Br J Cancer; 1999;80:1058-61.

134. Giovannucci E, et al. Intake of carotenoids and retinol in relation to risk of prostate cancer. J Natl Cancer Inst. 1995 Dec 6;87(23):1767-76.

135. Giovannucci E. Tomatoes, tomato-based products, lycopene, and cancer: review of the epidemiologic literature. J Natl Cancer Inst. 1999 Feb 17;91(4):317-31

136. Giri A, et al. Vitamin C mediated protection on cisplatin induced mutagenicity in mice. Mutat Res. 1998 Nov 3;421(2):139-48.

137. Glick JH, et al. Phase I clinical trials of WR-2721 with alkylating agent chemotherapy. Int J Radiat Oncol Biol Phys. 1982 Mar-Apr;8(3-4):575-80.

138. Gogos CA, et al. Dietary omega-3 polyunsaturated fatty acids plus vitamin E restore immunodeficiency and prolong survival for severely ill patients with generalized malignancy: a randomized control trial. Cancer. 1998 Jan 15;82(2): 395-402

139. Gogos CA, et al. The effect of dietary omega-3 polyunsaturated fatty acids on T-lymphocyte subsets of patients with solid tumors. Cancer Detect Prev. 1995;19(5):415-7.

140. Gol-Winkler R, et al. Ascorbic acid effect on methylcholanthrene-induced transformation in C3H10T1/2 clone 8 cells. Toxicology. 1980;17(2):237-9.

141. Gonzalez Flecha BS, et al. Inhibition of microsomal lipid peroxidation by alpha-tocopherol and alpha-tocopherol acetate. Xenobiotica. 1991 Aug;21(8):1013-22.

142. Gonzalez NJ, et al. Evaluation of pancreatic proteolytic enzyme treatment of adenocarcinoma of the pancreas, with nutrition and detoxification support. Nutr Cancer. 1999;33(2):117-24.

143. Graham S, et al. Dietary factors in the epidemiology of cancer of the larynx. Am J Epidemiol.

1981 Jun;113(6):675-80.

144. Greenberg ER, et al. A clinical trial of antioxidant vitamins to prevent colorectal adenoma. Polyp Prevention Study Group. N Engl J Med. 1994 Jul 21;331(3):141-7.

145. Gressier B, et al. Scavenging of reactive oxygen species by letosteine, a molecule with two blocked-SH groups. Comparison with free-SH drugs. Pharm World Sci. 1995 May 26;17(3): 76-80.

146. Gridley G, et al. Diet and Oral and Pharyngeal Cancer Among Blacks. Nutr Cancer 1990;14:219-225 (1990).

147. Groopman, JE and Itri, LM. Chemotherapy-induced anemia in adults: incidence and treatment. JNCI 1999;91:1616-1634.

148. Haenszel W, et al. Developments in the epidemiology of stomach cancer over the past decade. Cancer Res. 1975 Nov;35(11 Pt. 2):3452-9.

149. Hajarizadeh H, et al. Protective effect of doxorubicin in vitamin C or dimethyl sulfoxide against skin ulceration in the pig. Ann Surg Oncol. 1994 Sep;1(5):411-4.

150. Halliwell, B. Antioxidants and human disease: A general introduction. Nutr Rev 1997;55:S44-S52.

151. Han D, et al. Protection against glutamate-induced cytotoxicity in C6 glial cells by thiol antioxidants. Am J Physiol. 1997 Nov;273(5 Pt 2):R1771-8.

152. Hannemann J, et al. Cisplatin-induced lipid peroxidation and decrease of gluconeogenesis in rat kidney cortex: different effects of antioxidants and radical scavengers. Toxicology. 1988 Oct;51(2-3):119-32.

153. Hasebe M, et al. Glutamate in enteral nutrition: can glutamate replace glutamine in supplementation to enteral nutrition in burned rats? JPEN J Parenter Enteral Nutr. 1999 Sep-Oct;23(5 Suppl):S78-82.

154. Head KA. Ascorbic acid in the prevention and treatment of cancer. Altern Med Rev. 1998 Jun;3(3):174-86.

155. Hehr T, et al. [Role of sodium selenite as an adjuvant in radiotherapy of rectal carcinoma]. Med Klin. 1997 Sep 15;92 Suppl 3:48-9.

156. Heimann SW. Pycnogenol for ADHD? J Am Acad Child Adolesc Psychiatry. 1999 Apr;38(4):357-8.

157. Heinle RW and Welch, AD. Experiments with pteroylglutamic acid and pteroylglutamic acid deficiency in human leukemia. J Clin Invest 1948;27:539.

158. Henquin N, et al. Nutritional monitoring and counselling for cancer patients during chemotherapy. Oncology. 1989;46(3):173-7.

159. Henson DE, et al.Ascorbic acid: biologic functions and relation to cancer. J Natl Cancer Inst. 1991 Apr 17;83(8):547-50.

160. Herbert V, et al. Destruction of vitamin B12 by ascorbic acid. JAMA. 1974 Oct 14;230(2):241-2.

161. Herman EH, et al. Comparison of the effectiveness of (+/-)-1,2-bis(3,5-dioxopiperazinyl-1-yl)propane (ICRF-187) and N-acetylcysteine in preventing chronic doxorubicin cardiotoxicity in beagles. Cancer Res. 1985 Jan;45(1):276-81.

162. Herman EH, et al. Effect of pretreatment with ICRF-187 on the total cumulative dose of doxorubicin tolerated by beagle dogs. Cancer Res. 1988 Dec 1;48(23):6918-25.

163. Herman EH, et al. Pretreatment with ICRF-187 allows a marked increase in the total cumulative dose of doxorubicin tolerated by beagle dogs. Drugs Exp Clin Res. 1988;14(9):563-70.

164. Herman EH, et al. Reduction of chronic daunorubicin cardiotoxicity by ICRF-187 in rabbits. Res Commun Chem Pathol Pharmacol. 1981 Jan;31(1):85-97.

165. Herman EH, et al. Reduction of chronic doxorubicin cardiotoxicity in beagle dogs by bis-morpholinomethyl derivative of razoxane (ICRF-159). Cancer Chemother Pharmacol. 1987;19(4):277-81.

166. Herman EH, et al.Comparison of the effectiveness of (+/-)-1,2-bis(3,5-dioxopiperazinyl-1-yl)propane (ICRF-187) and N-acetylcysteine in preventing chronic doxorubicin cardiotoxicity in beagles. Cancer Res. 1985 Jan;45(1):276-81.

167. Herman EH, et al.Influence of vitamin E and ICRF-187 on chronic doxorubicin cardiotoxicity in miniature swine. Lab Invest. 1983 Jul;49(1):69-77.

168. Hida H, et al. Effect of antioxidants on adriamycin-induced microsomal lipid peroxidation. Biol Trace Elem Res. 1995 Jan-Mar;47(1-3):111-6.

169. Higginson, J. Etiological factors in gastro-intestinal cancer in man. J Natl Cancer Inst 1966;37:527-545.

170. Hirose M, et al. Inhibition of mammary gland carcinogenesis by green tea catechins and other naturally occurring antioxidants in female Sprague-Dawley rats pretreated with 7,12-dimethylbenz[alpha]anthracene. Cancer Lett. 1994 Aug 15;83(1-2):149-56.

171. Hodges S, et al. CoQ10: could it have a role in cancer management? Biofactors. 1999;9(2-4):365-70.

172. Hoefer-Janker H, et al. 1st clinical experience with subtoxic vitamin A doses during radiation and cytostatic tumor therapy. Krebsartz 1969;24(4):203-7.

172a. Hong WK, et al. Prevention of second primary tumors with isotretinoin in squamous-cell carcinoma of the head and neck. [see comments] N Engl J Med 1990;323:795-801.

173. Horton R. The new new public health of risk and radical engagement. Lancet. 1998 Jul 25;352(9124):251-2.

174. Howell A, et al. Inhibition of the adherence of P-fimbriated Escherichia coli to uroepithelial-cell surfaces by proanthocyanidin extracts from cranberries. N Engl J Med 1998 Oct 8;339(15):1085-6

175. Hussain SP and Rao AR. Chemopreventive action of selenium on methylcholanthrene-induced carcinogenesis in the uterine cervix of mouse. Oncology 1992;49(3):237-40.

176. Huynh HT, et al.Effects of intragastrically administered Pycnogenol on NNK metabolism in F344 rats. Anticancer Res. 1999 May-Jun;19(3A):2095-9.

177. Iarussi D, et al. Protective effect of coenzyme Q10 on anthracyclines cardiotoxicity: control study in children with acute lymphoblastic leukemia and non-Hodgkin lymphoma. Mol Aspects Med. 1994;15 Suppl:s207-12.

178. Ibric LL, et al.Mechanisms of ascorbic acid-induced inhibition of chemical transformation in C3H/10T1/2 cells. Am J Clin Nutr. 1991 Dec;54(6 Suppl):1236S-1240S.

179. Ip C, et al. Mammary cancer prevention by regular garlic and selenium-enriched garlic. Nutr

Cancer 1992;17(3):179-86.

180. Israel L, et al. [Vitamin A augmentation of the effects of chemotherapy in metastatic breast cancers after menopause. Randomized trial in 100 patients]. Ann Med Interne (Paris). 1985;136(7):551-4.et al.

181. Ito H, et al. Vitamin E prevents endothelial injury associated with cisplatin injection into the superior mesenteric artery of rats. Heart Vessels. 1995;10(4):178-84.

182. Jaffey M. Vitamin C and cancer: examination of the Vale of Leven trial results using broad inductive reasoning. Med Hypotheses. 1982 Jan;8(1):49-84.

183. Jang M, et al. Cancer chemopreventive activity of resveratrol, a natural product derived from grapes. Science. 1997 Jan 10;275(5297):218-20.

184. Jebb SA, et al. 5-fluorouracil and folinic acid-induced mucositis: no effect of oral glutamine supplementation. Br J Cancer. 1994 Oct;70(4):732-5.

185. Jensen GL, et al. A double-blind, prospective, randomized study of glutamine-enriched compared with standard peptide-based feeding in critically ill patients. Am J Clin Nutr. 1996 Oct;64(4):615-21.

186. Jiang XR, et al. The anti-leukaemic effects and the mechanism of sodium selenite. Leuk Res. 1992;16(4):347-52.

187. Johnston CS. Biomarkers for establishing a tolerable upper intake level for vitamin C. Nutr Rev. 1999 Mar;57(3):71-7.

188. Jolliet P, et al.Plasma coenzyme Q10 concentrations in breast cancer: prognosis and therapeutic consequences. Int J Clin Pharmacol Ther. 1998 Sep;36(9):506-9.

189. Joseph JA, et al. Reversals of age-related declines in neuronal signal transduction, cognitive, and motor behavioral deficits with blueberry, spinach, or strawberry dietary supplementation. J Neurosci. 1999 Sep 15;19(18):8114-21.

190. Julka D, et al. Adriamycin-induced oxidative stress in rat central nervous system. Biochem Mol Biol Int. 1993 Apr;29(5):807-20.

191. Kagerud A, et al. Influence of tocopherol on tumour cell oxygenation. Cancer Lett. 1978 Oct;5(4):185-9.

192. Kagerud A, et al. Tocopherol in irradiation of experimental neoplasms. Influence of dose and administration. Acta Radiol Oncol. 1981;20(2):97-100.

193. Kagerud A, et al. Tocopherol in irradiation of temporary hypoxic tumours. Acta Radiol Oncol. 1981;20(1):1-4.

194. Kallistratos G, et al. Inhibition of benzo(a)pyrene carcinogenesis in rats with vitamin C. J Cancer Res Clin Oncol. 1980;97(1):91-6.

195. Kamen BA, et al.Methotrexate accumulation and folate depletion in cells as a possible mechanism of chronic toxicity to the drug. Br J Haematol. 1981 Nov;49(3):355-60.

196. Karpov LM, et al. [Permeability of the mitochondrial membranes of the organs of white rats innoculated with Walker carcinoma to lipoic acid and thiamine labelled with S35]. Vopr Onkol. 1975;21(8):69-73.

197. Karpov LM, et al. [S35 lipoic acid distribution and its effect on pyruvate dehydrogenase activity in rats with Walker carcinoma]. Vopr Onkol. 1977;23(10):87-90. Russian.

198. Kaugars GE, et al. Use of antioxidant supplements in the treatment of human oral leukoplakia. Oral Surg Oral Med Oral Pathol Oral Radiol Endod. 1996 Jan;81(1):5-14.

199. Kawasaki N, et al. Cardiac energy metabolism at several stages of adriamycin-induced heart failure in rats. Int J Cardiol. 1996 Aug;55(3):217-25.

200. Kessler H, et al. Potential protective effect of vitamin C on carcinogenesis caused by nitrosamine in drinking water: an experimental study on Wistar rats. Eur J Surg Oncol. 1992 Jun;18(3):275-81.

201. Khachik F, et al. Lutein, lycopene, and their oxidative metabolites in chemoprevention of cancer. J Cell Biochem Suppl. 1995;22:236-46. 21

202. Khoss AE, et al. [L-carnitine therapy and myocardial function in children treated with chronic hemodialysis]. Wien Klin Wochenschr. 1989 Jan 6;101(1):17-20.

203. Kim JM, et al. Chemopreventive effects of carotenoids and curcumins on mouse colon carcinogenesis after 1,2-dimethylhydrazine initiation. Carcinogenesis. 1998 Jan;19(1):81-5.

204. Kishi T, et al. Bioenergetics in clinical medicine: prevention by forms of coenzyme Q of the inhibition by Adriamycin of coenzyme Q10-enzymes in mitochondria of the myocardium. Proc Natl Acad Sci U S A. 1976 Dec;73(12):4653-6.

205. Kishi T, et al. Letter: Prevention by coenzyme Q10 (NSC-140865) of the inhibition by Adriamycin (NSC-123127) of coenzyme Q10 enzymes. Cancer Treat Rep. 1976 Mar;60(3):223-4.

206. Klenner F.R. Virus pneumonia and its treatment with vitamin C. Southern Med Surgery., Feb. 1948.

207. Kligerman MM, et al. Interim analysis of a randomized trial of radiation therapy of rectal cancer with/without WR-2721. Int J Radiat Oncol Biol Phys. 1992;22(4):799-802.

208. Klimberg VS, et al. Claude H. Organ, Jr. Honorary Lectureship. Glutamine, cancer, and its therapy. Am J Surg. 1996 Nov;172(5):418-24.

209. Klimberg VS, et al. Glutamine suppresses PGE2 synthesis and breast cancer growth. J Surg Res. 1996 Jun;63(1):293-7.

210. Kolonel LN, et al. Association of diet and place of birth with stomach cancer incidence in Hawaii Japanese and Caucasians. Am J Clin Nutr. 1981 Nov;34(11):2478-85.

211. Komiyama S, et al. Synergistic combination therapy of 5-fluorouracil, vitamin A, and cobalt-60 radiation for head and neck tumors—antitumor combination therapy with vitamin A. Auris Nasus Larynx. 1985;12 Suppl 2:S239-43.

212. Komiyama S, et al. [Multidisciplinary treatment of the head and neck cancer—FAR therapy and its modification and application]. Gan To Kagaku Ryoho. 1986 Apr;13(4 Pt 2):1731-6. Japanese.

213. Koterov AN, et al. [The effect of zinc metallothionein on lipid peroxidation in rodent bone marrow cells]. Radiats Biol Radioecol. 1998 May-Jun;38(3):426-31

214. Kotoh S, et al. Metallothionein expression is correlated with cisplatin resistance in transitional cell carcinoma of the urinary tract. J Urol. 1994 Oct;152(4):1267-70.

215. Kovacikova Z, et al. The effect of graded ascorbic acid intake on the activity of GSH-Px in the liver of female guinea pigs. Z Ernahrungswiss.

1995 Sep;34(3):220-3.

216. Krishnaswamy K, et al. A case study of nutrient intervention of oral precancerous lesions in India. Eur J Cancer B Oral Oncol. 1995 Jan;31B(1):41-8.

217. Krivit W. Adriamycin cardiotoxicity amelioration by alpha-tocopherol. Am J Pediatr Hematol Oncol. 1979 Summer;1(2):151-3.

218. Kuratomi Y, et al. Comparison of survival rates of patients with nasopharyngeal carcinoma treated with radiotherapy, 5-fluorouracil and vitamin A ("FAR" therapy) vs FAR therapy plus adjunctive cisplatin and peplomycin chemotherapy. Eur Arch Otorhinolaryngol. 1999;256 Suppl 1:S60-3.

219. Kurbacher CM, et al. Ascorbic acid (vitamin C) improves the antineoplastic activity of doxorubicin, cisplatin, and paclitaxel in human breast carcinoma cells in vitro. Cancer Lett. 1996 Jun 5;103(2):183-9.

220. Kushi LH, et al. Intake of vitamins A, C, and E and postmenopausal breast cancer. The Iowa Women's Health Study. Am J Epidemiol. 1996 Jul 15;144(2):165-74.

221. La Vecchia C. Mediterranean epidemiological evidence on tomatoes and the prevention of digestive-tract cancers. Proc Soc Exp Biol Med. 1998 Jun;218(2):125-8.

222. Labriola D and Livingston R. Possible interactions between dietary antioxidants and chemotherapy. Oncology 1999;13:1003-11.

223. Ladner C, et al. Effect of etoposide (VP16-213) on lipid peroxidation and antioxidant status in a high-dose radiochemotherapy regimen. Cancer Chemother Pharmacol. 1989;25(3):210-2.

224. Lamm DL, et al. Megadose vitamins in bladder cancer: a double-blind clinical trial. J Urol 1994 Jan;151(1):21-6.

225. Laohavinij S, et al. A phase I clinical study of the antipurine antifolate lometrexol (DDATHF) given with oral folic acid. Invest New Drugs. 1996;14(3):325-35.

226. Laszlo, John. The Cure of Childhood Leukemia : Into the Age of Miracles. Rutgers University Press, 1996.

227. Lazo JS, et al. The protein thiol metallothionein as an antioxidant and protectant against antineoplastic drugs. Chem Biol Interact. 1998 Apr 24;111-112:255-62.

228. Le Marchand L, et al. Intake of specific carotenoids and lung cancer risk. Cancer Epidemiol Biomarkers Prev. 1993 May-Jun;2(3):183-7.

229. Lekili M, et al. Zinc plasma levels in prostatic carcinoma and BPH. Int Urol Nephrol. 1991;23(2):151-4.

230. Levine M, et al. Vitamin C pharmacokinetics in healthy volunteers: evidence for a recommended dietary allowance. Proc Natl Acad Sci U S A. 1996 Apr 16;93(8):3704-9.

231. Levine M, et al. Criteria and recommendations for vitamin C intake. JAMA. 1999 Apr 21;281(15):1415-23.

232. Levy J, et al. Lycopene is a more potent inhibitor of human cancer cell proliferation than either alpha-carotene or beta-carotene. Nutr Cancer. 1995;24(3):257-66.

233. Li JY, et al. [Preliminary report on the results of nutrition prevention trials of cancer and other common diseases among residents in Linxian, China].Chung Hua Chung Liu Tsa Chih. 1993 May;15(3):165-81.

234. Links M and Lewis C. Chemoprotectants: a review of their clinical pharmacology and therapeutic efficacy. Drugs 1999 Mar;57(3):293-308.Emphasis added.

235. Lissoni P, et al. A randomised study with subcutaneous low-dose interleukin 2 alone vs interleukin 2 plus the pineal neurohormone melatonin in advanced solid neoplasms other than renal cancer and melanoma. Br J Cancer. 1994 Jan;69(1):196-9.

236. Lissoni P, et al. A randomized study of chemotherapy with cisplatin plus etoposide versus chemoendocrine therapy with cisplatin, etoposide and the pineal hormone melatonin as a first-line treatment of advanced non-small cell lung cancer patients in a poor clinical state. J Pineal Res. 1997 Aug;23(1):15-9.

237. Lissoni P, et al. A randomized study of immunotherapy with low-dose subcutaneous interleukin-2 plus melatonin vs chemotherapy with cisplatin and etoposide as first-line therapy for advanced non-small cell lung cancer. Tumori. 1994 Dec 31;80(6):464-7.

238. Lissoni P, et al. A randomized study of neuroimmunotherapy with low-dose subcutaneous interleukin-2 plus melatonin compared to supportive care alone in patients with untreatable metastatic solid tumour. Support Care Cancer. 1995 May;3(3):194-7.

239. Lissoni P, et al. A randomized study with the pineal hormone melatonin versus supportive care alone in patients with brain metastases due to solid neoplasms. Cancer. 1994 Feb 1;73(3):699-701.

240. Lissoni P, et al. Biological and clinical results of a neuroimmunotherapy with interleukin-2 and the pineal hormone melatonin as a first line treatment in advanced non-small cell lung cancer. Br J Cancer. 1992 Jul;66(1):155-8.

241. Lissoni P, et al. Biotherapy with the pineal immunomodulating hormone melatonin versus melatonin plus aloe vera in untreatable advanced solid neoplasms. Nat Immun. 1998;16(1):27-33.

242. Lissoni P, et al. Chemoneuroendocrine therapy of metastatic breast cancer with persistent thrombocytopenia with weekly low-dose epirubicin plus melatonin: a phase II study. J Pineal Res. 1999 Apr;26(3):169-73.

243. Lissoni P, et al. Chemoneuroendocrine therapy of metastatic breast cancer with persistent thrombocytopenia with weekly low-dose epirubicin plus melatonin: a phase II study. J Pineal Res. 1999 Apr;26(3):169-73.

244. Lissoni P, et al. Increased survival time in brain glioblastomas by a radioneuroendocrine strategy with radiotherapy plus melatonin compared to radiotherapy alone. Oncology. 1996 Jan-Feb;53(1):43-6.

245. Lissoni P, et al. Is there a role for melatonin in the treatment of neoplastic cachexia? Eur J Cancer. 1996 Jul;32A(8):1340-3.

246. Lissoni P, et al. Subcutaneous therapy with low-dose interleukin-2 plus the neurohormone melatonin in metastatic gastric cancer patients with low performance status. Tumori. 1993 Dec 31;79(6):401-4.

247. Lissoni P, et al. Treatment of cancer chemotherapy-induced toxicity with the pineal hormone melatonin. Support Care Cancer. 1997 Mar;5(2):126-9.

248. Lissoni P, et al. A phase II study of tamoxifen plus melatonin in metastatic solid tumour patients. Br J Cancer. 1996 Nov;74(9):1466-8.

249. Lissoni P, et al. Modulation of cancer endocrine therapy by melatonin: a phase II study of tamoxifen plus melatonin in metastatic breast cancer patients progressing under tamoxifen alone. Br J Cancer. 1995 Apr;71(4):854-6.

250. Lissoni P, et al. Randomized study with the pineal hormone melatonin versus supportive care alone in advanced nonsmall cell lung cancer resistant to a first-line chemotherapy containing cisplatin. Oncology. 1992;49(5):336-9.

251. Liu FJ, et al. Pycnogenol enhances immune and haemopoietic functions in senescence-accelerated mice. Cell Mol Life Sci. 1998 Oct;54(10):1168-72.

252. Locatelli MC, et al. A phase II study of combination chemotherapy in advanced ovarian carcinoma with cisplatin and cyclophosphamide plus reduced glutathione as potential protective agent against cisplatin toxicity. Tumori. 1993 Feb 28;79(1):37-9.

253. Lockwood K, et al. Partial and complete regression of breast cancer in patients in relation to dosage of coenzyme Q10. Biochem Biophys Res Commun. 1994 Mar 30;199(3):1504-8.

254. Lockwood K, et al. Progress on therapy of breast cancer with vitamin Q10 and the regression of metastases. Biochem Biophys Res Commun. 1995 Jul 6;212(1):172-7.

255. Loehrer PJ Sr. The history of ifosfamide. Semin Oncol. 1992 Dec;19(6 Suppl 12):2-6.

256. Lu HZ, et al. Effects of beta-carotene on doxorubicin-induced cardiotoxicity in rats. Chung Kuo Yao Li Hsueh Pao. 1996 Jul;17(4):317-20.

256a. Lund, EL, et al. Oral ubiquinone intake reduces the in vivo radiosensitivity of human small cell lung cancer. Proc AACR Abstract #1664, 1997.

257. Luoma PV, et al. Serum selenium, glutathione peroxidase activity and high-density lipoprotein cholesterol—effect of selenium supplementation. Res Comm Chem Pathol Pharmacol. 1984 Dec;46(3):469-72.

258. Lupulescu A. Vitamin C inhibits DNA, RNA and protein synthesis in epithelial neoplastic cells. Int J Vitam Nutr Res. 1991;61(2):125-9.

259. Lupulescu A. Ultrastructure and cell surface studies of cancer cells following vitamin C administration. Exp Toxicol Pathol. 1992 Mar;44(1):3-9.

260. Ma J, et al. Methylenetetrahydrofolate reductase polymorphism, dietary interactions, and risk of colorectal cancer.Cancer Res. 1997 Mar 15;57(6):1098-102.

261. Malick MA, et al. Effect of vitamin E on post irradiation death in mice. Experientia. 1978 Sep 15;34(9):1216-7.

263. Mansur, DB, et al. Inhibition of Ras Mediated Transformation and Jun Kinase Activation by the Selenoorganic Compound Ebselen. Proc Annu Meet Am Soc Clin Oncol; 1999;18:A2454.

264. Marcus M, et al. Stability of vitamin B12 in the presence of ascorbic acid in food and serum: restoration by cyanide of apparent loss. Am J Clin Nutr. 1980 Jan;33(1):137-43.

265. Marcus SL, et al. Hypovitaminosis C in patients treated with high-dose interleukin 2 and lymphokine-activated killer cells. Am J Clin Nutr. 1991 Dec;54(6 Suppl):1292S-1297S.

266. Marcus SL, et al. Severe hypovitaminosis C occurring as the result of adoptive immunotherapy with high-dose interleukin 2 and lymphokine-activated killer cells. Cancer Res. 1987 Aug 1;47(15):4208-12.

267. Mathews-Roth MM. Antitumor activity of beta-carotene, canthaxanthin and phytoene. Oncology. 1982;39(1):33-7.

268. McCall MR, et al.Can antioxidant vitamins maternally reduce oxidative damage in humans? Free Radic Biol Med. 1999 Apr;26(7-8):1034-53.

269. McDonald S, et al. Preliminary results of a pilot study using WR-2721 before fractionated irradiation of the head and neck to reduce salivary gland dysfunction. Int J Radiat Oncol Biol Phys. 1994 Jul 1;29(4):747-54

270. McEligot AJ, et al. Comparison of serum carotenoid responses between women consuming vegetable juice and women consuming raw or cooked vegetables. Cancer Epidemiol Biomarkers Prev. 1999 Mar;8(3):227-31.

271. McKeown-Eyssen G, et al. A randomized trial of vitamins C and E in the prevention of recurrence of colorectal polyps. Cancer Res. 1988 Aug 15;48(16):4701-5.

272. Meadows GG, et al. Ascorbate in the treatment of experimental transplanted melanoma. Am J Clin Nutr. 1991 Dec;54(6 Suppl):1284S-1291S.

273. Mei W, et al. Study of immune function of cancer patients influenced by supplemental zinc or selenium-zinc combination. Biol Trace Elem Res. 1991 Jan;28(1):11-9.

274. Mehta MP. Protection of normal tissues from the cytotoxic effects of radiation therapy: focus on amifostine. Semin Radiat Oncol. 1998 Oct;8(4 Suppl 1):14-6.

275. Mehta, J. Intake of antioxidants among American cardiologists. Am J Cardiol. 1997 Jun 1;79(11):1558-60.

276. Meinsma, L. [Nutrition and Cancer]. Voeding 1964;25:357-365.

277. Memik F, et al. The etiological role of diet, smoking, and drinking habits of patients with esophageal carcinoma in Turkey. J Environ Pathol Toxicol Oncol. 1992 Jul-Aug;11(4):197-200.

279. Meydani M, et al. The effect of long-term dietary supplementation with antioxidants. Ann N Y Acad Sci. 1998 Nov 20;854:352-60.

280. Meydani M, et al. A closer look at vitamin E. Can this antioxidant prevent chronic diseases? Postgrad Med. 1997 Aug;102(2):199-201, 206-7.

281. Milas L, et al. Protective effects of S-2-(3-aminopropylamino) ethylphosphorothioic acid against radiation damage of normal tissues and a fibrosarcoma in mice. Cancer Res. 1982 May;42(5):1888-97.

282. Milei J, et al. Amelioration of adriamycin-induced cardiotoxicity in rabbits by prenylamine and vitamins A and E. Am Heart J. 1986 Jan;111(1):95-102.

283. Miller AL. Therapeutic considerations of L-Glutamine: a review of the literature. Altern Med Rev. 1999 Aug;4(4):239-248.

284. Mimnaugh EG, et al. The effects of alpha-tocopherol on the toxicity, disposition, and metabolism of adriamycin in mice. Toxicol Appl Pharmacol. 1979 Jun 15;49(1):119-26.

285. Mirvish SS, et al. Ascorbate-nitrite reaction: possible means of blocking the formation of carcinogenic N-nitroso compounds. Science. 1972 Jul

7;177(43):65-8.

286. Miyajima A, et al. N-acetylcysteine modifies cis-dichlorodiammineplatinum-induced effects in bladder cancer cells. Jpn J Cancer Res. 1999 May;90(5):565-70.

287. Mo H and Elson CE. Apoptosis and cell-cycle arrest in human and murine tumor cells are initiated by isoprenoids. J Nutr 1999 Apr;129(4): 804-13

288. Moertel CG, et al. High-dose vitamin C versus placebo in the treatment of patients with advanced cancer who have had no prior chemotherapy. A randomized double-blind comparison. N Engl J Med. 1985 Jan 17;312(3): 137-41.

289. Montilla P, et al. Antioxidative effect of melatonin in rat brain oxidative stress induced by Adriamycin. Rev Esp Fisiol. 1997 Sep;53(3): 301-5.

290. Montilla PL, et al. Oxidative stress in diabetic rats induced by streptozotocin: protective effects of melatonin. J Pineal Res. 1998 Sep;25(2):94-100.

291. Montilla P, et al. Hyperlipidemic nephropathy induced by adriamycin: effect of melatonin administration. Nephron. 1997;76(3):345-50.

292. Montilla PL, et al. Protective role of melatonin and retinol palmitate in oxidative stress and hyperlipidemic nephropathy induced by adriamycin in rats. J Pineal Res. 1998 Sep;25(2): 86-93.

293. Montilla P, et al. Protective role of melatonin and retinol palmitate in oxidative stress and hyperlipidemic nephropathy induced by adriamycin in rats. J Pineal Res. 1998 Sep;25(2):86-93.

294. Morgan SL, et al. Folic acid supplementation prevents deficient blood folate levels and hyperhomocysteinemia during longterm, low dose methotrexate therapy for rheumatoid arthritis: implications for cardiovascular disease prevention. J Rheumatol. 1998 Mar;25(3):441-6.

295. Morgan SL, et al. The effect of folic acid supplementation on the toxicity of low-dose methotrexate in patients with rheumatoid arthritis. Arthritis Rheum. 1990 Jan;33(1):9-18.

296. Morgan SL, et al. Supplementation with folic acid during methotrexate therapy for rheumatoid arthritis. A double-blind, placebo-controlled trial. Ann Intern Med. 1994 Dec 1;121(11): 833-41.

297. Morishima I, et al. Melatonin, a pineal hormone with antioxidant property, protects against adriamycin cardiomyopathy in rats. Life Sci. 1998;63(7):511-21.

298. Morishima I, et al. Zinc accumulation in adriamycin-induced cardiomyopathy in rats: effects of melatonin, a cardioprotective antioxidant. J Pineal Res. 1999 May;26(4):204-10.

299. Morishima I, et al. Zinc accumulation in adriamycin-induced cardiomyopathy in rats: effects of melatonin, a cardioprotective antioxidant. J Pineal Res. 1999 May;26(4):204-10

300. Morita M, et al. A new method to determine the level of coenzyme Q10 in one drop of human blood for biomedical research. Biochem Biophys Res Commun. 1993 Mar 31;191(3):950-4.

301. Morrow CS and Cowan KH. Drug resistance and its clinical circumvention. In: Holland JF, et al. Cancer Medicine, 4th Ed., Baltimore: Williams & Wilkins, 1997.

302. Moyad MA, et al. Vitamin E, alpha- and gamma-tocopherol, and prostate cancer. Semin Urol Oncol 1999 May;17(2):85-90

303. Muscaritoli M, et al. Oral glutamine in the prevention of chemotherapy-induced gastrointestinal toxicity. Eur J Cancer. 1997 Feb;33(2):319-20.

304. Myers CE, et al. Adriamycin: amelioration of toxicity by alpha-tocopherol. Cancer Treat Rep. 1976 Jul;60(7):961-2.

305. Myers CE, et al. Adriamycin: the role of lipid peroxidation in cardiac toxicity and tumor response. Science. 1977 Jul 8;197(4299):165-7.

306. Nakagawa M, et al. Potentiation by vitamin A of the action of anticancer agents against murine tumors. Jpn J Cancer Res. 1985 Sep;76(9):887-94.

307. Nakashima T, et al. Induction of apoptosis in maxillary sinus cancer cells by 5-fluorouracil, vitamin A and radiation (FAR) therapy. Eur Arch Otorhinolaryngol. 1999;256 Suppl 1:S64-9.

308. Narisawa T, et al. Inhibitory effects of natural carotenoids, alpha-carotene, beta-carotene, lycopene and lutein, on colonic aberrant crypt foci formation in rats. Cancer Lett. 1996 Oct 1;107(1):137-42.

309. Negri E, et al. Intake of selected micronutrients and the risk of breast cancer. Int J Cancer 1996;65:140-144 (1996).

310. Negri E, et al. Intake of selected micronutrients and the risk of endometrial carcinoma. Cancer 1996;77:917-923.

311. Neri B, et al. Differences between carnitine derivatives and coenzyme Q10 in preventing in vitro doxorubicin-related cardiac damages. Oncology. 1988;45(3):242-6.

312. Neri B, et al. Protective effect of L-carnitine on cardiac metabolic damage induced by doxorubicin in vitro. Anticancer Res. 1986 Jul-Aug;6(4):659-62.

313. Nesaretnam K, Stephen R, Dils R, Darbre P. Tocotrienols inhibit the growth of human breast cancer cells irrespective of estrogen receptor status.Lipids 1998 May;33(5):461-9.

314. Nesbitt JA, et al. Adriamycin-vitamin E combination therapy for treatment of prostate adenocarcinoma in the Nb rat model. J Surg Oncol. 1988 Aug;38(4):283-4.

315. Newmark HL, et al. Ascorbic acid and vitamin B12. JAMA. 1979 Nov 23;242(21):2319-20.

316. Newmark HL, et al. Stability of vitamin B12 in the presence of ascorbic acid. Am J Clin Nutr. 1976 Jun;29(6):645-9.

317. Nishino H. Cancer prevention by carotenoids. Mutat Res. 1998 Jun 18;402(1-2):159-63.

318. Noda Y, et al. Hydroxyl and superoxide anion radical scavenging activities of natural source antioxidants using the computerized JES-FR30 ESR spectrometer system. Biochem Mol Biol Int. 1997 Jun;42(1):35-44.

319. Nomura AM, et al. Serum vitamin levels and the risk of cancer of specific sites in men of Japanese ancestry in Hawaii. Cancer Res 1985;45:2369-2372.

320. Noto V, et al. Effects of sodium ascorbate (vitamin C) and 2-methyl-1,4-naphthoquinone (vitamin K3) treatment on human tumor cell growth in vitro. I. Synergism of combined vitamin C and K3 action. Cancer. 1989 Mar 1;63(5):901-6.

321. Ohhara H, et al. A protective effect of coenzyme

Q10 on the Adriamycin-induced cardiotoxicity in the isolated perfused rat heart. J Mol Cell Cardiol. 1981 Aug;13(8):741-52.

322. Ohnuma, Takoa, Anorexia and cachexia. In: Holland, JF, et al. Cancer Medicine, 4th Ed., Baltimore: Williams and Wilkins, 1997.

323. Ohshima H and Bartsch H. Chronic infections and inflammatory processes as cancer risk factors: possible role of nitric oxide in carcinogenesis. Mutat Res 1994 Mar 1;305(2):253-64

324. Okuma K, et al. [Protective effect of coenzyme Q10 in cardiotoxicity induced by Adriamycin]. Gan To Kagaku Ryoho. 1984 Mar;11(3):502-8.

325. Okunieff P, et al. Toxicity, radiation sensitivity modification, and combined drug effects of ascorbic acid with misonidazole in vivo on FSaII murine fibrosarcomas. J Natl Cancer Inst. 1987 Aug;79(2):377-81.

326. Okunieff P. Interactions between ascorbic acid and the radiation of bone marrow, skin, and tumor. Am J Clin Nutr. 1991 Dec;54(6 Suppl):1281S-1283S.

327. Okuno SH, et al. Phase III controlled evaluation of glutamine for decreasing stomatitis in patients receiving fluorouracil (5-FU)-based chemotherapy. Am J Clin Oncol. 1999 Jun;22(3):258-61.

328. Olafson RW. Intestinal metallothionein: effect of parenteral and enteral zinc exposure on tissue levels of mice on controlled zinc diets. J Nutr. 1983 Feb;113(2):268-75.

329. Omenn GS. Chemoprevention of lung cancer: the rise and demise of beta-carotene. Annu Rev Public Health. 1998;19:73-99.

330. Oomah, BD, et al. Microwave heating of grapeseed: effect on oil quality. J. Agric. Food Chem. 1998;456(10):4017-4021.

331. Oriana S, et al. A preliminary clinical experience with reduced glutathione as protector against cisplatin-toxicity. Tumori. 1987 Aug 31;73(4): 337-40.

332. Ormstad K, et al. Pharmacokinetics and metabolism of sodium 2-mercaptoethanesulfonate in the rat. Cancer Res. 1983 Jan;43(1):333-8.

333. Pack, George T. and Livingston, Edward M. Treatment of cancer and allied diseases. 3 vols. New York, NY: Paul B. Hoeber, 1940.

334. Packer L, et al. Alpha-lipoic acid: a metabolic antioxidant and potential redox modulator of transcription. Adv Pharmacol. 1997;38:79-101.

335. Packer L and C Coleman, The Antioxidant Miracle. New York: Wiley, 1999.

336. Packer L, et al. Antioxidant activity and biologic properties of a procyanidin-rich extract from pine (Pinus maritima) bark, pycnogenol. Free Radic Biol Med. 1999 Sep;27(5-6):704-24.

337. Paganelli G, et al. Effects of vitamins A, C, and E supplementation on rectal cell proliferation in patients with colorectal adenomas. J Natl Cancer Inst 1992;84:47-51.

338. Pakdaman A. Symptomatic treatment of brain tumor patients with sodium selenite, oxygen, and other supportive measures. Biol Trace Elem Res. 1998 Apr-May;62(1-2):1-6.

339. Palan PR, et al. Plasma Levels of Antioxidant Beta-Carotene and Alpha-Tocopherol in Uterine Cervix Dysplasias and Cancer. Nutr Cancer 1991;15:13-20.

340. Park JS, et al. Dietary lutein absorption from marigold extract is rapid in BALB/c mice. J Nutr. 1998 Oct;128(10):1802-6.

341. Park JS, et al. Dietary lutein from marigold extract inhibits mammary tumor development in BALB/c mice. J Nutr. 1998 Oct;128(10):1650-6.

342. Parovichnikova EN, et al. [Effectiveness of trans-retinoic acid in the treatment of acute promyelocytic leukemia: initial results of a multicenter study]. Ter Arkh. 1999;71(7):20-4.

343. Passwater, Richard A. All about antioxidants. Garden City Park: Avery, 1998.

344. Patt, HN, et al. Cysteine protection against irradiation. Science 1949;110:213.

345. Perez, Carlos A and Brady, Luther W., Principles and Practice of Radiation Oncology, Third Edition, Philadelphia: Lippincott-Raven, 1998.

346. Peto R, et al. Can dietary beta-carotene materially reduce human cancer rates? Nature. 1981 Mar 19;290(5803):201-8.

347. Pieri C, et al. Melatonin: a peroxyl radical scavenger more effective than vitamin E. Life Sci. 1994;55(15):PL271-6.

348. Pierson HF, et al. Modulation of peroxidation in murine melanoma by dietary tyrosine-phenylalanine restriction, levodopa methylester chemotherapy, and sodium ascorbate supplementation. J Natl Cancer Inst. 1985 Sep;75(3): 507-16.

349. Pierson HF, et al. Sodium ascorbate enhancement of carbidopa-levodopa methyl ester antitumor activity against pigmented B16 melanoma. Cancer Res. 1983 May;43(5):2047-51.

350. Pierson HF, et al.Influence of supplemental ascorbate on the antitumor activity of 5-hydroxydopa, a purported cytotoxic metabolite. Cancer Lett. 1985 Nov;29(2):157-68.

351. Pieters JJ. Nutritional teratogens: a survey of epidemiological literature. Prog Clin Biol Res. 1985;163B:419-29.

352. Pieters R, et al. Cytotoxic effects of vitamin A in combination with vincristine, daunorubicin and 6-thioguanine upon cells from lymphoblastic leukemic patients. Jpn J Cancer Res. 1991 Sep;82(9):1051-5.

353. Podmore ID, et al. Vitamin C exhibits pro-oxidant properties. Nature. 1998 Apr 9;392(6676):559.

354. Potischman N, et al. Breast cancer and dietary and plasma concentrations of carotenoids and vitamin A. Am J Clin Nutr 1990; 52:909-915.

355. Powell-Tuck J, et al. A double blind, randomized, controlled trial of glutamine supplementation in parenteral nutrition. Gut. 1999 Jul;45(1):82-8.

356. Powis G, et al. Doxorubicin-induced hair loss in the Angora rabbit: a study of treatments to protect against the hair loss. Cancer Chemother Pharmacol. 1987;20(4):291-6.

357. Prasad KN, et al. High doses of multiple antioxidant vitamins: essential ingredients in improving the efficacy of standard cancer therapy. J Am Coll Nutr. 1999 Feb;18(1):13-25.

358. Prasad KN, et al. Cancer prevention studies: past, present, and future directions. Nutrition. 1998 Feb;14(2):197-210

359. Prasad KN, et al. Modification of the effect of tamoxifen, cis-platin, DTIC, and interferon-alpha 2b on human melanoma cells in culture by a mixture of vitamins. Nutr Cancer. 1994;22(3):233-45.

360. Prasad KN, et al. Sodium ascorbate potentiates the growth inhibitory effect of certain agents on

neuroblastoma cells in culture. Proc Natl Acad Sci USA. 1979 Feb;76(2):829-32.

361. Prasad MP, et al. Micronuclei and carcinogen DNA adducts as intermediate end points in nutrient intervention trial of precancerous lesions in the oral cavity. Eur J Cancer B Oral Oncol. 1995 May;31B(3):155-9.

362. Prasad SB, et al. Use of subtherapeutical dose of cisplatin and vitamin C against murine Dalton's lymphoma. Pol J Pharmacol Pharm. 1992 Jul-Aug;44(4):383-91.

363. Protasov DA, et al. [The role of cardioxane (ICRF-187) in the prevention of cardiotoxicity of anthracyclines in the combined drug therapy of extensive ovarian cancer]. Vopr Onkol. 1998;44(6):718-21.

364. Przybyszewski WM, et al. Protection against hydroxyurea-induced cytotoxic effects in L5178Y cells by free radical scavengers. Cancer Lett. 1982 Nov-Dec;17(2):223-8.

365. Przybyszewski WM, et al. Protection of L5178Y cells by vitamin E against acute hydroxyurea toxicity does not change the efficiency of ribonucleotide reductase-mediated hydroxyurea-induced cytotoxic events. Cancer Lett. 1987 Mar;34(3):337-44.

366. Rana K, et al. Radioprotection of chick thymus by vitamin E. Indian J Exp Biol. 1993 Oct;31(10):847-9.

367. Rapozzi V, et al. Melatonin and oxidative damage in mice liver induced by the prooxidant antitumor drug, adriamycin. In Vivo. 1999 Jan-Feb;13(1):45-50.

368. Rapozzi V, et al. Effects of melatonin administration on tumor spread in mice bearing Lewis lung carcinoma. Pharmacol Res. 1992 Feb-Mar;25 Suppl 1:71-2.

369. Rapozzi V, et al.Melatonin decreases bone marrow and lymphatic toxicity of adriamycin in mice bearing TLX5 lymphoma. Life Sci. 1998;63(19):1701-13.

370. Rautalahti MT, et al. The effects of supplementation with alpha-tocopherol and beta-carotene on the incidence and mortality of carcinoma of the pancreas in a randomized, controlled trial. Cancer. 1999 Jul 1;86(1):37-42.

371. Recchia F, et al. Beta-interferon, retinoids and tamoxifen combination in advanced breast cancer. Clin Ter. 1998 May-Jun;149(3):203-8.

372. Reddy BS, et al. Chemoprevention of colon carcinogenesis by the synthetic organoselenium compound 1,4-phenylenebis(methylene)selenocyanate. Cancer Res 1992;52(20):5635-40.

372a. Reichman M, et al. Serum vitamin A and subsequent development of prostate cancer in the first national health and nutrition examination survey epidemiologic follow-up study. Cancer Research 1990;50:2311-2315.

373. Richardson, MA, et al. Alternative/complementary medicine: implications for patient-provider communication. Proc Annu Meet Am Soc Clin Oncol; 1999;18:A2279.

374. Ripoll EA, et al. Vitamin E enhances the chemotherapeutic effects of adriamycin on human prostatic carcinoma cells in vitro. J Urol. 1986 Aug;136(2):529-31.

375. Romanenko VI. [Melatonin as a possible endogenous leukemogenic (blastomogenic) agent]. Gematol Transfuziol. 1983 Feb;28(2):47-50.

376. Rong Y, et al. Pycnogenol protects vascular endothelial cells from t-butyl hydroperoxide induced oxidant injury. Biotechnol Ther. 1994-95;5(3-4):117-26.

377. Roosen N, et al. Effect of pharmacologic doses of zinc on the therapeutic index of brain tumor chemotherapy with carmustine. Cancer Chemother Pharmacol. 1994;34(5):385-92.

378. Rosin MP, et al.The effect of ascorbate on 3-methylcholanthrene-induced cell transformation in C3H/10T1/2 mouse-embryo fibroblast cell cultures. Mutat Res. 1980 Aug;72(3):533-7.

379. Rostock RA, et al. Evaluation of high-dose vitamin E as a radioprotective agent. Radiology. 1980 Sep;136(3):763-6.

380. Rouse K, et al. Glutamine enhances selectivity of chemotherapy through changes in glutathione metabolism. Ann Surg. 1995 Apr;221(4):420-6.

381. Rubio IT, et al. Effect of glutamine on methotrexate efficacy and toxicity. Ann Surg. 1998 May;227(5):772-8; discussion 778-80.

382. Rybak LP, et al. Dose dependent protection by lipoic acid against cisplatin-induced ototoxicity in rats: antioxidant defense system. Toxicol Sci. 1999 Feb;47(2):195-202.

382a. Saffiotti U. Role of vitamin A in carcinogenesis. Am J Clin Nutr 1969 Aug;22(8):1088.

383. Saiag P, et al. Treatment of early AIDS-related Kaposi's sarcoma with oral all-trans-retinoic acid: results of a sequential non-randomized phase II trial. Kaposi's Sarcoma ANRS Study Group. Agence Nationale de Recherches sur le SIDA. AIDS. 1998 Nov 12;12(16):2169-76.

384. Salasche SJ, et al. Clinical pearl: vitamin E (alpha-tocopherol), 800 IU daily, may reduce retinoid toxicity. J Am Acad Dermatol. 1999 Aug;41(2 Pt 1):260.

385. Samoilov AV, et al. [The radioprotective and antioxidant properties of solubilized alpha-tocopherol acetate]. Eksp Klin Farmakol. 1992 Jul-Aug;55(4):42-4.

386. Santos MS, et al. Beta-carotene-induced enhancement of natural killer cell activity in elderly men: an investigation of the role of cytokines. Am J Clin Nutr. 1998 Jul;68(1): 164-70.

387. Sarkar SR, et al. Effect of whole body gamma radiation on reduced glutathione contents of rat tissues. Strahlentherapie. 1983 Jan;159(1):32-3.

388. Sarma L, et al. Protective effects of vitamins C and E against gamma-ray-induced chromosomal damage in mouse. IRB. 1993 Jun;63(6):759-64.

389. Satoh M, et al. Modulation of resistance to anticancer drugs by inhibition of metallothionein synthesis. Cancer Res. 1994 Oct 15;54(20):5255-7.

390. Savvov VI, et al. [Pyruvate oxidation and S35-lipoic acid fixation by breast tumor homogenates]. Vopr Onkol. 1978;24(8):97-9.

391. Sawada H, et al. [Chronic cardiotoxicity of Adriamycin and the possible prevention by coenzyme Q10 in rabbits]. Nippon Gan Chiryo Gakkai Shi. 1979 Apr 20;14(2):143-51.

392. Sayed-Ahmed MM, et al. Reversal of doxorubicin-induced cardiac metabolic damage by L-carnitine. Pharmacol Res. 1999 Apr;39(4): 289-95.

393. Scheef W, et al. Controlled clinical studies with an antidote against the urotoxicity of oxazaphosphorines: preliminary results. Cancer Treat Rep. 1979 Mar;63(3):501-5.

394. Schilsky RL. Methotrexate: An Effective Agent

for Treating Cancer and Building Careers. The Polyglutamate Era. Oncologist. 1996;1(4): 244-247.

394a. Schloerb PR, et al. Total parenteral nutrition with glutamine in bone marrow transplantation and other clinical applications (a randomized, double-blind study). JPEN J Parenter Enteral Nutr. 1993 Sep-Oct;17(5):407-13.

395. Schrauzer GN, et al. Effect of simulated American, Bulgarian, and Japanese human diets and of selenium supplementation on the incidence of virally induced mammary tumors in female mice. Biol Trace Elem Res. 1989 Apr-May;20(1-2):169-78.

396. Schroder H, et al. Folic acid supplements in vitamin tablets: a determinant of hematological drug tolerance in maintenance therapy of childhood acute lymphoblastic leukemia. Pediatr Hematol Oncol. 1986;3(3):241-7.

397. Schwartz JL, et al. Beta-carotene and/or vitamin E as modulators of alkylating agents in SCC-25 human squamous carcinoma cells. Cancer Chemother Pharmacol. 1992;29(3):207-13.

398. Schwartz JL. The dual roles of nutrients as antioxidants and prooxidants: their effects on tumor cell growth. J Nutr. 1996 Apr;126(4 Suppl):1221S-7S.

399. Scott DL, et al. The influence of dietary selenium and vitamin E on glutathione peroxidase and glutathione in the rat. Biochim Biophys Acta. 1977 Mar 29;497(1):218-24.

400. Sen CK, et al. Regulation of cellular thiols in human lymphocytes by alpha-lipoic acid: a flow cytometric analysis. Free Radic Biol Med. 1997;22(7):1241-57.

401. Shaheen AA, et al. Radioprotection of whole-body gamma-irradiation-induced alteration in some haematological parameters by cysteine, vitamin E and their combination in rats. Strahlenther Onkol. 1991 Aug;167(8):498-501.

402. Shamberger RJ and Rudolph G. Protection against cocarcinogenesis by antioxidants. Experientia. 1966 Feb 15;22(2):116

403. Shamberger RJ, et al. Antioxidants and cancer. Part VI. Selenium and age-adjusted human cancer mortality. Arch Environ Health. 1976 Sep-Oct;31(5):231-5.

404. Shichiri M, et al. Apparent low levels of ubiquinone in rat and human neoplastic tissues. Int Z Vitaminforsch. 1968;38(5):472-81.

405. Shimpo K, et al. Ascorbic acid and adriamycin toxicity. Am J Clin Nutr. 1991 Dec;54(6 Suppl):1298S-1301S.

406. Shinozawa S, et al. Effect of high dose alpha-tocopherol and alpha-tocopherol acetate pretreatment on adriamycin (doxorubicin) induced toxicity and tissue distribution. Physiol Chem Phys Med NMR. 1988;20(4):329-35.

407. Shug AL. Protection from adriamycin-induced cardiomyopathy in rats. Z Kardiol. 1987;76 Suppl 5:46-52.

408. Sieja K. Selenium (Se) deficiency in women with ovarian cancer undergoing chemotherapy and the influence of supplementation with this micro-element on biochemical parameters. Pharmazie. 1998 Jul;53(7):473-6.

409. Simon JA, et al. Relation of serum ascorbic acid to serum vitamin B12, serum ferritin, and kidney stones in U.S. adults. Arch Intern Med. 1999 Mar 22;159(6):619-24.

410. Simon JA, et al. Relationship of ascorbic acid to blood lead levels. JAMA. 1999 Jun 23-30;281(24):2289-93.

411. Singh LR, et al. Effect of whole body gamma-radiation on glutathione reductase of rat tissues. Strahlenther Onkol. 1987 May;163(5):337-9.

412. Singh VN, et al. Premalignant lesions: role of antioxidant vitamins and beta-carotene in risk reduction and prevention of malignant transformation. Am J Clin Nutr. 1991 Jan;53(1 Suppl):386S-390S.

413. Sinha R, et al. Organic and inorganic selenium compounds inhibit mouse mammary cell growth in vitro by different cellular pathways. Cancer Lett. 1996 Oct 22;107(2):277-84.

414. Skibola CF, et al. Polymorphisms in the methylenetetrahydrofolate reductase gene are associated with susceptibility to acute leukemia in adults. Proc Natl Acad Sci U S A. 1999 Oct 26;96(22):12810-12815.

415. Skubitz KM, et al. Oral glutamine to prevent chemotherapy induced stomatitis: a pilot study. J Lab Clin Med. 1996 Feb;127(2):223-8.

416. Souba WW, et al. Glutamine nutrition in the management of radiation enteritis. JPEN J Parenter Enteral Nutr. 1990 Jul-Aug;14(4 Suppl):106S-108S.

417. Souba WW. Glutamine and cancer. Ann Surg. 1993 Dec;218(6):715-28.

418. Speek,-A.J.; Schrijver,-J.; Schreurs,-W.H.P. J-Food-Sci. Chicago, Ill. : Institute of Food Technologists. Jan/Feb 1985. v. 50 (1) p. 121-124.

419. Spirichev VB, et al. [The effect of administration of beta-carotene in an oil solution on its blood serum level and antioxidant status of patients with duodenal ulcer and erosive gastritis]. Vopr Med Khim. 1992 Nov-Dec;38(6):44-7.

420. Srinivasan V, et al. Radioprotection by vitamin E: injectable vitamin E administered alone or with WR-3689 enhances survival of irradiated mice. Int J Radiat Oncol Biol Phys. 1992;23(4):841-5.

421. Steinach G, et al. Vitamin A supplements, fried foods, fat and urothelial cancer, a case-referrant study in Stockholm in 1985-1987. International Journal of Cancer 1990;45:1006-11.

422. Stratford MR, et al. Studies on the role of antioxidants in radioprotection. Pharmacol Ther. 1988;39(1-3):389-91

423. Strauss M, et al. Carnitine promotes heat shock protein synthesis in adriamycin-induced cardiomyopathy in a neonatal rat experimental model. J Mol Cell Cardiol. 1998 Nov;30(11):2319-25.

424. Studer UE, et al. Adjuvant treatment with a vitamin A analogue (etretinate) after transurethral resection of superficial bladder tumors. Final analysis of a prospective, randomized multicenter trial in Switzerland. Eur Urol. 1995;28(4):284-90.

425. Sturniolo GC, et al. Zinc therapy increases duodenal concentrations of metallothionein and iron in Wilson's disease patients. Am J Gastroenterol. 1999 Feb;94(2):334-8.

426. Subar AF, et al. Fruit and vegetable intake in the United States: the baseline survey of the Five A Day for Better Health Program. Am J Health Promot. 1995 May-Jun;9(5):352-60.

427. Subramaniam S, et al. Vitamin E protects intestinal basolateral membrane from CMF-induced

damages in rat. Indian J Physiol Pharmacol. 1995 Jul;39(3):263-6.

428. Sukolinskii VN, et al. [Prevention of postoperative complications in patients with stomach cancer using an antioxidant complex]. Vopr Onkol. 1989;35(10):1242-5.

429. Sundstrom H, et al. Serum selenium and glutathione peroxidase, and plasma lipid peroxides in uterine, ovarian or vulvar cancer, and their responses to antioxidants in patients with ovarian cancer. Cancer Lett. 1984 Aug;24(1):1-10.

430. Sundstrom H, et al. Supplementation with selenium, vitamin E and their combination in gynaecological cancer during cytotoxic chemotherapy. Carcinogenesis. 1989 Feb;10(2):273-8.

431. Suzuki KT, et al. Production of hydroxyl radicals by copper-containing metallothionein: roles as prooxidant. Toxicol Appl Pharmacol. 1996 Nov;141(1):231-7.

432. Svingen BA, et al. Protection against adriamycin-induced skin necrosis in the rat by dimethyl sulfoxide and alpha-tocopherol. Cancer Res. 1981 Sep;41(9 Pt 1):3395-9.

433. Svingen BA, et al. Protection by alpha-tocopherol and dimethylsulfoxide (DMSO) against adriamycin induced skin ulcers in the rat. Res Commun Chem Pathol Pharmacol. 1981 Apr;32(1):189-92.

434. Synold TW, et al. Antineoplastic activity of continuous exposure to dexrazoxane: potential new role as a novel topoisomerase II inhibitor. Semin Oncol. 1998 Aug;25(4 Suppl 10):93-9.

435. Szczepannska I, et al. Amelioration of hydroxyurea-induced suppression of phagocytosis in human granulocytes by free radical scavengers. Scand J Haematol. 1985 Jan;34(1):35-8.

436. Szczepanska I, et al. Inhibition of leucocyte migration by cancer chemotherapeutic agents and its prevention by free radical scavengers and thiols. Eur J Haematol. 1988 Jan;40(1):69-74.

437. Tanaka Y and Sugahara T. Clinical experiences of chemical radiation protection in tumor radiotherapy in Japan.In: Brady LW, ed. Radiation Sensitizers, p. 421. New York: Masson, 1980.

438. Tanigawa N, et al. Effect of vitamin E on toxicity and antitumor activity of adriamycin in mice. Jpn J Cancer Res. 1986 Dec;77(12):1249-55.

439. Taper HS, et al. Non-toxic potentiation of cancer chemotherapy by combined C and K3 vitamin pre-treatment. Int J Cancer. 1987 Oct 15;40(4):575-9.

440. Taper HS, et al. Non-toxic sensitization of cancer chemotherapy by combined vitamin C and K3 pretreatment in a mouse tumor resistant to oncovin. Anticancer Res. 1992 Sep-Oct;12(5):1651-4.

441. Taper HS, et al. Potentiation of radiotherapy by nontoxic pretreatment with combined vitamins C and K3 in mice bearing solid transplantable tumor. Anticancer Res. 1996 Jan-Feb;16(1):499-503.

442. Tavares DC, et al. Protective effects of the amino acid glutamine and of ascorbic acid against chromosomal damage induced by doxorubicin in mammalian cells. Teratog Carcinog Mutagen. 1998;18(4):153-61.

443. Taylor PR, et al. Prevention of esophageal cancer: the nutrition intervention trials in Linxian, China. Linxian Nutrition Intervention Trials Study Group. Cancer Res. 1994 Apr 1;54(7 Suppl):2029s-2031s.

444. Teicher BA, et al. In vivo modulation of several anticancer agents by beta-carotene. Cancer Chemother Pharmacol. 1994;34(3):235-41.

445. Tesoriere L, et al. Effect of vitamin A administration on resistance of rat heart against doxorubicin-induced cardiotoxicity and lethality. J Pharmacol Exp Ther. 1994 Apr;269(1):430-6.

446. Thiruvengadam R,, et al. Effect of antioxidant vitamins and mineral on chemotherapy induced cytopenia. Proc Annu Meet Am Soc Clin Oncol; 1996;15:A1793.

447. Turrisi AT, et al. Final report of the phase I trial of single-dose WR-2721 [S-2-(3-aminopropylamino)ethylphosphorothioic acid]. Cancer Treat Rep. 1986 Dec;70(12):1389-93.

448. Umegaki K, et al. Decrease in vitamin E levels in the bone marrow of mice receiving whole-body X-ray irradiation. Free Radic Biol Med. 1994 Nov;17(5):439-44.

449. Umegaki K, et al. Increases in 4-hydroxynonenal and hexanal in bone marrow of rats subjected to total body X-ray irradiation: association with

450. Umegaki K, et al. Whole body X-ray irradiation to mice decreases ascorbic acid concentration in bone marrow: comparison between ascorbic acid and vitamin E. Free Radic Biol Med. 1995 Oct;19(4):493-7.

451. Usui T, et al. Possible prevention from the progression of cardiotoxicity in Adriamycin-treated rabbits by coenzyme Q10. Toxicol Lett. 1982 Jun;12(1):75-82.

452. Vadhanavikit S, et al. Micro-analysis for coenzyme Q10 in endomyocardial biopsies of cardiac patients and data on bovine and canine hearts. Biochem Biophys Res Commun. 1984 Sep 28;123(3):1165-9.

453. van den Berg H. Effect of lutein on beta-carotene absorption and cleavage. Int J Vitam Nutr Res. 1998;68(6):360-5.

454. van het Hof KH, et al.Bioavailability of lutein from vegetables is 5 times higher than that of beta-carotene. Am J Clin Nutr. 1999 Aug;70(2):261-8.

455. Van Zandwijk, U. Randomized trial of chemoprevention with vitamin A and N-acetylcysteine in patients with cancer of the upper and lower airways: the Euroscan study. Proc Annu Meet Am Soc Clin Oncol; 1999;18:A1788.

456. Vanella A, et al.Enhanced resistance of adriamycin-treated MCR-5 lung fibroblasts by increased intracellular glutathione peroxidase and extracellular antioxidants. Biochem Mol Med. 1997 Oct;62(1):36-41.

457. Varga JM, et al. Inhibition of transplantable melanoma tumor development in mice by prophylactic administration of Ca-ascorbate. Life Sci. 1983 Apr 4;32(14):1559-64.

458. Venturini M, et al.Multicenter randomized controlled clinical trial to evaluate cardioprotection of dexrazoxane versus no cardioprotection in women receiving epirubicin chemotherapy for advanced breast cancer. J Clin Oncol. 1996 Dec;14(12):3112-20.

459. Verastegui E, et al. A natural cytokine mixture (IRX-2) and interference with immune suppression induce immune mobilization and regression of head and neck cancer. Int J Immunopharmacol. 1997 Nov-Dec;19(11-12):619-27.

459a. Veronesi U, et al. Randomized trial of fenretinide to prevent second breast malignancy in women with early breast cancer. J Natl Ca Inst

1999 Nov 3;91(21):1847-56.

460. Vile GF, et al. Microsomal lipid peroxidation induced by adriamycin, epirubicin, daunorubicin and mitoxantrone: a comparative study. Cancer Chemother Pharmacol. 1989;24(2):105-8

461. Villani F, et al. Effect of glutathione and N-acetylcysteine on in vitro and in vivo cardiac toxicity of doxorubicin. Free Radic Res Commun. 1990;11(1-3):145-51.

462. Virgili F, et al. Procyanidins extracted from Pinus maritima (Pycnogenol): scavengers of free radical species and modulators of nitrogen monoxide metabolism in activated murine RAW 264.7 macrophages. Free Radic Biol Med. 1998 May;24(7-8):1120-9.

463. Waalkes MP, et al. Effect of chronic dietary zinc deficiency on cadmium toxicity and carcinogenesis in the male Wistar [Hsd: (WI)BR] rat. Toxicol Appl Pharmacol. 1991 May;108(3):448-56.

464. Warrell, Raymond P, Jr. Differentiation Agents. In: DeVita, VT, et al. Cancer: Principles & Practice of Oncology, 5th Ed., Philadelphia: Lippincott-Raven, 1997.

465. Washburn LC, et al. Distribution of WR-2721 in normal and malignant tissues of mice and rats bearing solid tumors: dependence on tumor type, drug dose and species. Radiat Res. 1974 Aug;59(2):475-83.

466. Wassertheil-Smoller S, et al. Dietary vitamin C and uterine cervical dysplasia. Am J Epidemiol. 1981 Nov;114(5):714-24.

467. Watne, AL, et al. The diagnosis and surgical treatment of patients with Gardner's syndrome. Surgery 1977;82:327-333.

468. Waxman S, et al. The enhancement of 5-fluorouracil anti-metabolic activity by leucovorin, menadione and alpha-tocopherol. Eur J Cancer Clin Oncol. 1982 Jul;18(7):685-92.

469. Weijl NI, et al. Cisplatin combination chemotherapy induces a fall in plasma antioxidants of cancer patients. Ann Oncol. 1998 Dec;9(12):1331-7.

470. White WS, et al. The ferret as a model for evaluation of the bioavailabilities of all-trans-beta-carotene and its isomers. J Nutr. 1993 Jun;123(6):1129-39.

471. Willett WC, et al. Prediagnostic serum selenium and risk of cancer. Lancet. 1983 Jul 16;2(8342):130-4.

472. Williamson JM, et al. Intracellular cysteine delivery system that protects against toxicity by promoting glutathione synthesis. Proc Natl Acad Sci U S A. 1982 Oct;79(20):6246-9.

473. Wood LA. Possible prevention of adriamycin-induced alopecia by tocopherol. N Engl J Med. 1985 Apr 18;312(16):1060.

474. Woodson K, et al. Serum alpha-Tocopherol and Subsequent Risk of Lung Cancer Among Male Smokers. J Natl Cancer Inst. 1999 Oct 20;91(20):1738-1743.

475. Xu ZL, et al. [Detoxifying effect of lisheng-se on cisplatin and its relation to metallothionein induction]. Chung Hua Chung Liu Tsa Chih. 1994 Jul;16(4):280-3.

475a. Xu ZL, et al. [The effect of zinc glycyrrhizate on toxicity and anticancer activity of cisplatin in mice]. Yao Hsueh Hsueh Pao. 1993;28(8):567-71.

476. Xue KX, et al. Comparative studies on genotoxicity and antigenotoxicity of natural and synthetic beta-carotene stereoisomers. Mutat Res. 1998 Oct 12;418(2-3):73-8.

477. Yasukawa M, et al. Radiation-induced neoplastic transformation of C3H10T1/2 cells is suppressed by ascorbic acid. Radiat Res. 1989 Dec;120(3):456-67.

478. Yeum, K., et al. Beta-carotene intervention trial in premalignant gastric lesions. Journal of the American College of Nutrition, 995;14:536:A48.

479. Yu SY, et al. Protective role of selenium against hepatitis B virus and primary liver cancer in Qidong. Biol Trace Elem Res. 1997 Jan;56(1):117-24.

480. Zhang S, et al. A prospective study of folate intake and the risk of breast cancer. JAMA. 1999 May 5;281(17):1632-7.

481. Zhang S, et al. Dietary carotenoids and vitamins A, C, and E and risk of breast cancer. J Natl Cancer Inst. 1999 Mar 17;91(6):547-56.

482. Zhang Z, et al. Uptake and distribution of sodium selenite in rat brain tumor. Biol Trace Elem Res. 1995 Apr;48(1):45-50.

483. Zheng W, et al. Retinol, Antioxidant Vitamins and Cancers of Upper Digestive Tract in a Prospective Cohort Study of Postmenopausal Women. Am J Epidemiol 1995;142:955-960.

484. Ziegler RG, et al. Does beta-carotene explain why reduced cancer risk is associated with vegetable and fruit intake? Cancer Res. 1992 Apr 1;52(7 Suppl):2060s-2066s.

485. Ziegler TR, et al. Clinical and metabolic efficacy of glutamine-supplemented parenteral nutrition after bone marrow transplantation. A randomized, double-blind, controlled study. Ann Intern Med. 1992 May 15;116(10):821-8.

486. Zima T, et al. ICRF-187 (dexrazoxan) protects from adriamycin-induced nephrotic syndrome in rats. Nephrol Dial Transplant. 1998 Aug;13(8):1975-9.

487. Zimmermann JS, et al. Pharmacological management of acute radiation morbidity. Strahlenther Onkol. 1998 Nov;174 Suppl 3:62-5.

Other Books by Ralph W. Moss, Ph.D.

Cancer Therapy: The Independent Consumer's Guide to Non-Toxic Treatment & Prevention

You want the full story on non-toxic treatment and prevention, and that's exactly what this landmark book delivers. *Cancer Therapy* is a must for cancer patients and their families who want: practical information on the most promising, non-toxic treatments; scientific evidence in readable language; well documented resource lists and medical references. Author Ralph W. Moss, Ph.D. has been called "possibly the best science writer in our midst" and "a revolutionary in the war on cancer."
$19.95 528 pp trade paperback Equinox Press

Herbs Against Cancer

History and Controversy

Herbs Against Cancer is the first comprehensive guide to the use of herbs in preventing and treating cancer. Ralph Moss has thoroughly explored the most important areas in this contentious field. He explores the most potent anti-cancer herbs and their uses, and offers both practical guidelines as well as the intriguing background of this subject. The links between herbalism and modern chemotherapy are made clear. This book is popularly written for people who seek to be involved and informed about their health care. The book has been critically acclaimed by leaders in the field of medicinal herbalism.
$16.95 216 pp trade paperback Equinox Press

The Cancer Industry

The Classic Exposé on the Cancer Establishment

This book shows why the billion dollar war on cancer is going nowhere. It details how drug companies influence cancer policy, how major industries keep the emphasis away from prevention, how the establishment maintains a blacklist of unconventional practitioners, and how the government has collaborated in the suppression of new ideas.
$16.95 528 pp. trade paperback Equinox Press

Questioning Chemotherapy

Finally, a powerful and intelligent critique of chemotherapy! This up-to-date book from acclaimed medical writer Ralph W. Moss, Ph.D. probes the scientific and statistical evidence to reveal the shocking truth: chemotherapy is inappropriate, ineffective and, in fact, dangerous for most of the people who receive it. Yet up to 600,000 Americans every year get chemo at their doctor's recommendation.

"A masterpiece of global importance in the history of medicine."
—Hans Nieper, MD,
Past Pres., German Society of Oncology

$19.95 214 pp trade paperback Equinox Press

Alternative Medicine Online
A Guide To Natural Remedies On the Internet

The Perfect Guide to the Best Alternative Health Sites Online. This special book directs the reader "off the beaten path" to a wealth of information on health and healing. With his trademark blend of clarity, wit, and common sense, Ralph Moss explores the most useful, intriguing. and sometimes off-beat sites in cyberspace. Second Edition, 1999. Organizes information in a visually appealing, easy to use format. Entertains while it educates with its wry observations and witty style. Directs readers to hard-to-find sites they'll love to explore. Puts the fascinating world of alternative medicine at their fingertips

$12.95 205 pp trade paperback Equinox Press